Alzheimer's Unmasked

Paul A. Barton

authorHOUSE®

AuthorHouse™
1663 Liberty Drive, Suite 200
Bloomington, IN 47403
www.authorhouse.com
Phone: 1-800-839-8640

First published by AuthorHouse 3/17/2008

ISBN: 978-1-4343-1823-7 (sc)
ISBN: 978-1-4343-5990-2 (hc)

Printed in the United States of America
Bloomington, Indiana

This book is printed on acid-free paper.

www..zapalzheimers.com

Contents

Disclaimer

I am not a medical doctor. I have no degrees. What I have is a twelve year self education in investigating the things involved in Alzheimer's disease. I also have no laboratory. My body has been my testing laboratory. It is not my intention to give medical advice to you. My intent here is to share with you the things I have learned. You should present this information to your doctor for his or her consideration. He or she has the legal authority to prescribe treatment for Alzheimer's disease, I do not.

Also, very importantly, to those of you in the medical field who have published, **I want to say Thank You.** This has allowed me to learn from you. I do not know anyone I have more respect and admiration for than people in medicine and neuroresearch.

Acknowledging
Our Creator

I want to acknowledge our Creator, for his *"miracle gift"* and for his *"guidance."* Without his help, I could not have succeeded.

As the author of this book, I am only the messenger, just another sinner trying to do better.

This book is a true testimonial as to the magnificent intelligence of our Creator, and his ability to inspire.

When we pray to our Creator, we must stay vigilant, lest our prayers are answered, but we be left unaware.

Dedication

To Mother

Mildred Juanita Gosman Barton

Taken from us by the Alzheimer's disease

May 16, 1999

Research
And
Review

The book titled, *Every Writer's Guide to Copyright And Publishing Law, says,* "Sometimes you can use a work without permission even if it is protected by copyright, provided your use falls within the parameters of "fair use." *The book goes on to say,* "The U.S. Copyright Law allows the reproduction, distribution, and adaptation of copyrighted material if the use is for purposes such as criticism, comment, news reporting, teaching, or research." I believe this book meets these requirements.

Alzheimer's is a horrible disease. It robs people of their dignity and steals their memory. I invite you to review with me the following research and teachings of the things involved in Alzheimer's disease. If you have never seen what Alzheimer's disease can do to a person's brain, I invite you to visit an Alzheimer's care facility. There, you will witness first hand how this disease is destroying people's minds, and bringing anxiety and grief to helpless family members.

Alzheimer's disease must be stopped.

I hope that our combined effort can bring this dementia under control or better yet, to end it completely.

PRESIDENT RONALD REAGAN

Why did President Ronald Reagan develop Alzheimer's disease? Two things we know, he loved jelly beans so much he kept a jar of them on his desk also he loved to eat ice cream in the evenings.

Both jelly beans and ice cream contain the chemicals of strong oxidizers. These can cause oxidation of metalloproteins in the elderly, thereby, inhibiting an enzymes ability to rapidly catalyze biochemical reactions.

In my opinion, his memory problems started as certain atomic elements in his body became oxidized. His memory problems showed up as his body became deficient in certain vitamins and atomic elements.

That is the reason why when a clinical trial is held, regarding certain chemicals in our diet, they will not show up as a problem until the memory starts to fail. Memory will weaken as the vitamin and element deficiency increases. This is one reason this mysterious disease has been so hard to unravel.

My findings are that certain chemicals in our diet require two things to trigger memory deficit, an elderly body and a weakened biochemical system.

Younger people's memory may not be affected by these chemicals because their biochemical systems are still strong.

Technical information

I am sure you are aware that Alzheimer's dementia is a very complicated disease. Any book that would attempt to explain it would contain a lot of technical information. If you don't enjoy the challenge of reading technical information I would advise you to skip over it and read what you understand. I wrote Chapter 16 titled "To The Point" especially for you. I believe it contains the information you are looking for.

In Chapter 17 Titled Conclusion "Putting It All Together" I use published neuroscience research to prove that the "6 numbers" [6 elements] are definitely involved in Alzheimer's dementia.

A LETTER

This is a copy of a letter I sent to three major Pharmaceutical companies, in an effort to help stop Alzheimer's disease. Two years has passed and I have not heard one word in reply. All three of these companies are looking for a cure for Alzheimer's disease.

Go figure.

Note: If any one of these three companies would have replied to my letter, I would have been glad to tell them that x and y represented certain chemicals in our diet.

11/4/2005

Dear Doctor _____,

I have been researching Alzheimer's disease [AD] going on 12 years now. Three years ago, I discovered how to reverse this disease in myself.

My work shows the pathogenesis of sporadic AD, to be based on element inhibition. The mechanisms that inhibit in biosynthesis are two combined substances, available worldwide. For now, let's call them X and Y.

Let me provide an example of what I am talking about. Although there are, multiple mechanisms involved in AD, [in excess of six] let's look at one, the low energy metabolism in the AD brain.

As you know, the Krebs cycle needs oxygen, supplied by the heme molecule. If we look at the molecular complex of the heme molecule, we find an iron atom at the center, bound to four nitrogen atoms.

Cliffs AP Biology 2nd Edition, page 75, states regarding anaerobic respiration that, "What if oxygen is not present? If oxygen is not present, there is no electron acceptor to accept the electrons at the end of the electron transport chain. If this occurs, then NADH accumulates. Once all the NAD+ has been converted to NADH, the Krebs cycle and Glycolysis both stop" [both need NAD+ to accept electrons.] "Once this happens, no new ATP is produced and the cell soon dies."

Combined X and Y inhibits the function of the nitrogen and iron atoms resulting in reduced cellular energy and eventually, the cells death.

Inhibited nitrogen atoms would also result in nitrogen deficiency, manifesting the waste and destruction of tissue, setting the stage for inflammation. Enter the need for non-inflammatory drugs. [Nsaids.]

Inhibited nitrogen atoms would also mean compromised amino acids and proteins like the mutated amino acid tryptophan, the precursor of niacin and serotonin. For serotonin, think selective serotonin reuptake inhibitors [SSRI.] For niacin think nutrition and choline for the acetylcholine neurotransmitter.

In my opinion, removing Abeta 1-42 peptide will not totally reverse AD because; inhibition of certain elements will remain. I believe that is why Elan Pharmaceuticals AN 1792, failed in clinical trials. In their mouse models, there was probably no inhibition of elements relating to AD.

Mother died of Alzheimer's disease in 1999, and shortly there after, AD symptoms started on me, just like they did on Mom.

Testing on myself, using a process of elimination, over a three year period, I was able to isolate X and Y. Then knowing the cause of my cognitive impairment, I was able to induce advanced symptoms normally not seen until early in the severe stage.

I then was able to totally reverse AD. The formula of numbers was responsible. Three times, I completed this alternating testing on myself, over a three-year time span. Each time one complete cycle took about six months. Each time the results were positive. Total restoration of memory and cognition.

I understand the following;

Why, in one study, statins reduced the onset of Alzheimer's dementia [AD] by 79%?

Why, two drinks a day of alcohol is AD protective?

Why, there is a connection between obesity and the higher risk of AD. [Mediterranean diet study?]

My formula may render Namenda [Memantine] and Aricept [Donepezil hydrochloride] obsolete, because, they cannot reverse Alzheimer's disease.

When I can find someone to produce this formula of numbers, then we can start to restore memory? This formula is a win-win situation. It can be used as both a diagnostic tool to determine who is at risk of AD, and as a therapy to restore cognition.

I am enclosing International Neuroscience Research abstracts on iron, heme, and nitrogen that support my findings. If your company has an interest in pursuing this, please contact me. I would like to help in ending this disease.

Sincerely,

_____

_____

INTRODUCTION
UNLOCKING THE MYSTERY OF ALZHEIMER'S

"HAS ANYONE TOLD YOU WHAT IS CAUSING THIS DISEASE, OR …WHAT MAY REVERSE IT?"

I want to share with you what I have learned from my years of private Alzheimer's research.

My research, including the testing on myself and information received from others, shows me that dementia can be stopped in its tracks, by doing nothing more then removing certain chemicals from the elderly persons diet, that is causing this problem.

At around age 65, I became at risk for sporadic Alzheimer's dementia, because my biochemical system had started to weaken from aging. Next, the ingesting of *"two combined chemicals,"* gradually began causing me cognitive impairment and dementia, by inhibiting certain *"atomic elements,"* I needed from my diet. The more of these *"two combined chemicals,"* I ingested, the more profound my memory problems became, as I grew older.

An Alzheimer's care facility would not have solved my problem because, there, I would have continued to ingest these *"two combined chemicals"* weekly, until many of my brain cells would have deteriorated, ceased to function and then died.

By continually replacing the *"atomic elements,"* that had been inhibited by the *"two combined chemicals,"* my memory improved. If, these *"atomic elements"* had not been replaced, my memory would be completely destroyed. This is what happened to my mother's memory. She died from full blown Alzheimer's disease. Now at age 72, my cognition and memory are normal again.

A diet that eliminates these chemicals is also necessary. [This is one reason the Mediterranean diet reduces the risk of Alzheimer's because, it does not contain any of these chemicals.] Another reason this diet reduces the risk of Alzheimer's is because it is supplying the 6 atomic elements that is needed for memory and cognition, plus vitamins.

There are several ways to treat a disease in the human body. Two of these are medicine and surgery. A third way is by naturopathy.

Stedman's Medical Dictionary, describes Naturopathy as, "A system of therapeutics in which neither surgical nor medicinal agents are used, with dependence being placed only on natural remedies." What we are talking about here is replacing atomic elements in my body that have lost their ionic [electrical] functions.

The element replacement has worked for me. Will it work for others? Common sense dictates that all of our bodies function biochemically in the same manner, which is the interaction of atomic elements, each with an ionic [electric] charge.

Let me explain, in order for a thought to proceed in my mind, an impulse must propagate itself down the entire length of the polarized membrane [nerve cell.] This is made possible as multiple sites along the nerve cell are de-polarized and re-polarized. When this occurs the electrical charge goes from a negative 70 milli-volts [mv] to a positive 35 mv. In this instance, if the sodium ions [$Na+$] have no ionic charge, depolarization stalls and the thought is lost.

When I refer to the ionic charge of atomic elements, keep in mind that sodium is one example of this. *Degussa Health and Nutrition Facts states,* "Life is essentially nothing more than a variety of biochemical reactions that occur continuously in the body." So, it should be obvious, if an atomic element is inhibited then the biochemical system in my body will not function properly, until it has been replaced.

I believe this Alzheimer's affliction has been misnamed. Instead of calling it Alzheimer's disease, I think a more accurate name would be "Alzheimer's deficiency."

Simply put, I believe that my cognitive decline was based upon a deficiency of "six atomic elements" that are needed to maintain my healthy mind and body.

My normal cognition has been completely restored by replacing these "six atomic elements" on a continual basis as needed?

Each of the other medications currently available to treat Alzheimer's, treats only a separate individual mechanism.

For example Namenda, [memantine HCl] marketed by Forest Laboratories, was recently approved on October 16, 2004, by the FDA to treat Alzheimer's. It works by blocking the build up of glutamate in the cell.

Another Alzheimer's medication is Aricept [Donepezil hydrochloride] approved for use November 26, 1996, and marketed by Pfizer Pharmaceutical Company. It is widely in use and acts as a cholinesterase inhibitor. This increases the effectiveness of the acetylcholine neurotransmitter.

Statins are also available to treat Alzheimer's. They work to reduce cholesterol by inhibiting a key enzyme involved in cholesterol production and can possibly reduce inflammation.

Information from the *American Academy of Neurology, [AAN] and published in Newswire, titled "Statin Drugs May Lower Risk of Alzheimer's."*

Dr. Robert C. Green et al., of Boston University School of Medicine says, "That their study confirms that taking statins was associated with a 79-percent reduction in the risk of developing Alzheimer's disease."

April 2002

The web site Alzheimerssupport.com relates that, "Statins block the vasoconstrictive effect of the A-beta protein." *Dr. Daniel Paris, lead author of the study at the University of South Florida, [USF] is an Assistant Professor at the USF Roskamp Institute, Dr. Paris relates that,* "These drugs appear to have anti-inflammatory properties also."

Alzheimerssupport.com says, "Recent studies have shown the risk of developing Alzheimer's disease is reduced in people treated with statins, however, the reason for this remains unclear."

The point I want to make here is this. If you look at the chemical formula in the literature that comes with two of the most effective statins, namely Crestor and Lipitor, what you will find is that two of the atomic elements in both of these medications are fluorine [atomic # 9] and nitrogen [atomic # 7.]

These statins are providing atomic element replacement therapy by replacing the inhibited atomic elements, fluorine and nitrogen. Crestor and Lipitor fend off Alzheimer's disease but cannot totally reverse the disease. Is this because, these two statins lack the other four atomic elements?

Further proof is evident when we look at the statin Zocor, distributed by Merck Pharmaceutical Company. Zocor was not performing as well as Crestor and Lipitor in clinical studies. So what did Merck do to compete? Guess what? Merck, combined Zocor with Vytorin, called it 10/10, 10/20, 10/40, 10/80 and now it is as effective as Crestor and Lipitor. Why is it effective? Because, Vytorin also contains fluorine and nitrogen. Vytorin is now a supped up version of Zocor.

Let's look at Pravachol, [pravastatin sodium] the third most effective statin. When we look at the empirical formula of Pravachol we find it contains sodium [atomic number 11.] Pravachol is replacing the atomic element sodium, another element that is inhibited in my brain.

SODIUM:

I knew there was a sodium deficiency in my brain from testing it on myself, but, in my years of research, I have not once read of any research on sodium deficiency in Alzheimer's. Imagine my surprise when my friend Pat told me her ex-husband passed away from Alzheimer's disease, and his doctor told her that her ex-husband had a severe sodium deficiency.

Sodium is number 11 in the *"Periodic Table of Atomic Elements."*

None of these three statin drugs will reverse the Alzheimer's disease. Is this because they do not contain the other three atomic elements? Treating myself with all *"six atomic elements"* restored my memory.

Based on research, my cognitive decline came about when these *"six atomic elements"* become electrically static, [atoms that have lost their ionic electrical charge.] Replacement therapy worked for me by replacing the *"six inhibited atomic elements,"* with *"six atomic elements"* that are ionic [atoms with an electric charge.]

My mother is buried under six feet of dirt back in Indiana, because no one knew how to stop her Alzheimer's disease. As the years went by, Mother's condition grew worse. All the while I was trying to understand what causes Alzheimer's and how to stop the progression. However, I just had too much to learn, and by the time I figured it all out Mother had been dead six years.

By replacing the *"six numbers,"* [atomic elements] on a continual basis, I was able to reverse the memory deficit in myself.

Five of the *"six atomic elements"* are approved safe for over the counter sales. The element fluorine is not approved for over the counter, but, the sub-unit fluoride is. A word of caution, not all trace elements and mineral supplements contain these six ionic charged atomic elements. More information is available on our web site at **www.zapalzheimers. com**

4

CHAPTER ONE:
INFORMATION AND STATISTICS

According to an article published in the, *Houston and Southwest Texas Chapter of the Alzheimer's Association, and written by Richard Taylor Ph.D.* "One neurologist stated that 95% of the people he diagnoses with Alzheimer's are not even tested. The patients, most of whom are in their mid to late 70s, would not be able to understand the instructions, let alone answer the questions, in a reliable manner."

Gabrielle Strobel of the Alzheimer's Research Forum interviewed, Vincent Marchesi in the online published forum, updated 11 July 2003.

The web page relates that, "Alzforum scientific advisor, Vincent Marchesi is currently director of the Boyer Center of Molecular Medicine at Yale University School of Medicine. When his wife, a doctor herself, was diagnosed with Alzheimer's disease eight years ago Marchesi developed an abiding interest in AD research." [AD is the abbreviation for Alzheimer's disease.]

Dr. Marchesi, who is also a pathologist, said, "I don't want to sound like an old fogy, but one of the problems in the daily reality of doing science nowadays is keeping track of what others have done. We are doing a huge amount of experimental work in many areas, and much of it is going unnoticed in the sense that it isn't being used by people other than those who actually make the observations. This is a mistake."

I believe Dr. Marchesi is correct. As extremely bright as the researchers are, for the most part each team is working on their particular project and I don't believe the left hand is completely aware of all of the information the right hand has.

What I have been doing for over seven years, practically day and night, seven days a week, is reading everything I could get my hands on pertaining to Alzheimer's dementia, in an effort to educate myself to as many things as possible that are involved in this disease. Since I didn't have an educational foundation for this, playing catch up has been tough, especially loading all that information into an old brain which at times, made recall fuzzy, if not impossible. The fact that Alzheimer's dementia was trying to take over my memory and cognition didn't help any. On the bad days I made do, and on the good days I made progress.

According to the following Alzheimer's web site,
http://www.downtownagusta.com/alzheimersstatistics.htm,
"Alzheimer's disease ranks fourth in the cause of deaths among adults. It is estimated that by the year 2025, there will be 34 million people world wide with dementia. Possibly, 60% of this number will suffer from Alzheimer's disease. Alzheimer's disease [AD] is a progressive, degenerative disease of the brain, and the most common form of dementia." The site further says, "Approximately 5 million Americans have Alzheimer's. Half of all nursing home residents suffer from AD or a related disorder. The average cost for nursing home care is $42,000 per year but can exceed $70,000 per year in some areas of the country. One person in ten over age 65 and nearly half over age 85 have Alzheimer's dementia, and a few people in there 30s and 40s have the disease. After onset of this disease, a person can expect to live from between 8 years to as long as 20 years." This is very depressing news. The web site further states, "14 million Americans will have AD by the middle of the next century unless a cure or prevention is found. The average lifetime cost per patient is $174,000. U. S. society spends at least $100 billion a year on AD. Neither Medicare, nor most private health insurance covers the long-term care most patients need."

Very large sums of money have been invested to find a cure for this disease. The above web site says, "The Alzheimer's Association has issued research grants for $185 million dollars to over 1200 projects." The U. S. Government spent over $ 400 million dollars on Alzheimer's research in one year. "By the year 2025, over 198,000 people in Georgia will have AD."

The Alzheimer's Association reports that, "By 2025, California will lead the nation with 820,000 people with the fatal brain disorder. Florida will have 712,000 with the disease, followed by Texas with 552,000. New York will have about 431,000. It is estimated that Pennsylvania will have 349,000 affected. Ohio is projected to have 308,000 people affected by Alzheimer's."

The U.K. web site http://www.Alz.co.uk/alzwp.htm relates that, "The number of people with dementia is rising quickly. By 2025, there will be four times the number of people with dementia in the developing world as there were in 1980. By 2025, 71% of all the people with dementia will be in developing countries." According to Alzheimer's Disease International, regarding a cure, the site says, "In the absence of effective prevention or treatment, the increase in the numbers of people with dementia will come about as a simple consequence of an increase in the size of the population most at risk. i.e., those aged 60 years and over."

Studies indicate taking estrogen replacement does not slow the progression of mild to moderate Alzheimer's disease in elderly women. There are several new drugs in the pipeline waiting for FDA approval, but nothing to cure the disease. They will only help to extend memory function. One class of drugs on the market that reduce inflammation is called Non-steroidal anti-inflammatory drugs [Nsaid's.]

Dr. Elwood Cohen makes the following comments on Nsaid's in his book, titled, "Alzheimer's Disease" regarding the nonprescription synthetic drugs that are available as anti-inflammatory products. He states that, "Some of these are, Motrin/Advil [Ibuprofen] with a recommended dosage of 200 mg, three to four times daily." *Dr. Cohen, says,* "They provide as much as 60 percent protection against Alzheimer's when started early in the course of the disease, because they retard the progression to dementia." *He further states that,* "Naproxen and Aleve are examples of other over-the-counter anti-inflammatory products, available and suggested at over-the-counter strengths. Side effects are, stomach distress bleeding ulcers. Inflammation of the liver and kidneys are potential problems although much less frequent are lower, over-the-counter strength."

Diet plays a major role in the prevention of Alzheimer's disease, as I will discuss in later chapters.

CHAPTER TWO:
WHAT IS
ALZHEIMER'S DEMENTIA?

In 1906, a German Neuropathologist, by the name of Alois Alzheimer diagnosed the first case. This dementia, was there after given the name, "Alzheimer's Disease."

The South Central Texas Chapter of the Alzheimer's Association answers, "What is dementia?" They say that, "Dementia is the loss of intellectual functions, such as thinking, remembering and reasoning of sufficient severity to interfere with a person's daily functioning." There are other cognitive impaired diseases also. The Alzheimer's Association goes on to say, "Some of the more well-known diseases that produce dementia include Alzheimer's disease, Multi-infarct dementia, Huntington's disease, Pick's disease, Creutzfeldt-Jakob disease and Parkinson's disease."

The Alzheimer's Association states in one of their publications that, "Significant memory loss is not a normal part of aging, and Alzheimer's can affect people as young as thirty."

The Alzheimer's Association also posts comments on the, "Ten warning signs you should know." They say, they are, "Memory loss, difficulty performing familiar tasks, problems with language, disorientation to time and place, poor or decreased judgment, exhibiting poor judgment about money, problems with abstract thinking, misplacing things, changes in mood or behavior, changes in personality and loss of initiative."

Here is one example of what it feels like when a person is suffering with Alzheimer's dementia, and having trouble thinking progressively. Suppose as a person with Alzheimer's, you walked through your kitchen and noticed dirty dishes in the sink. You would probably think, I need to wash those dishes, so you would turn the water on, but didn't remember you were supposed to close the drain with the stopper not to mention that you never added any dish detergent. Next, thinking about something else, you walk off and out of the room, leaving the water running. After awhile, when you came back through the kitchen you noticed the water was running. Not remembering you were just at the sink a few minutes ago, you might think, what is the water running for I'd better turn it off, never remembering, you were going to wash the dishes.

Not being able to think progressively is another one of the devastating effects of Alzheimer's dementia.

In my opinion, because of my age-weakened immune and biochemical defense system, my body could no longer process out certain chemical additives in my food and drink. When this occurred, I became at risk for Alzheimer's. Although, my body processed these combined chemical additives in my food and drink, all my life, with no problems. When I approached 65 years of age, my body stopped processing these combined chemical additives that were in my food and drink. This then, began causing me problems with my memory.

Cognitive function declined and synaptic transmission started to break down because brain cells and brain fibers became coated with a dissolved protein called beta amyloid plaque. This condition inhibits the acetylcholine neurotransmitter from carrying the message from the pre-synaptic nerve cell terminal across the space between the nerve cells called the synapse and received by the post synaptic nerve cell receptor.

As time goes by and more plaque is formed, there is more cognitive decline until eventually memory stops and the person loses the ability to speak because he or she can't access memory anymore to make or understand words. Medical science feels mutated enzymes gone amok causes this. So what are enzymes?

Stedman's Medical Dictionary describes an Enzyme as, "Any of numerous proteins or conjugated proteins produced by living organisms and functioning as specialized catalysts for biochemical reactions."

Some people in there 90's have no memory problems. It is obvious to me, that these people's bodies will still process these combined chemical food and drink additives.

Alzheimer's patients like my mother, who are placed in an Alzheimer's care facility, continue to build more amyloid plaque in their brain. Their condition continues to deteriorate because, in my opinion, the people working there unknowingly continue to feed them the very same chemical additives in food and drink that their bodies can no longer process.

Have you ever seen an Alzheimer's patient walk out of an Alzheimer's care facility cured? Mother's Alzheimer's condition continued to worsen until death came. She died a very undignified death. I felt so sorry for her, because no one knew how to stop this horrible disease. Until now there has been no known cause or termination of this disease. I want to bring my research to the attention of the neuro researchers and the twelve million people worldwide who are suffering from Alzheimer's dementia with little or no hope.

The sole reason I am writing this book is to share it directly with those families afflicted by this horrible disease. They should consult their doctor regarding this information.

I am beginning to understand why this mystery has existed for so long. There are so many different things involved. For one thing, a lot of the studies conflict and this causes confusion. In my opinion, based on years of private research, chemical additives in food and drink when combined are responsible for my cognitive impairment, dementia and memory loss because of my age weakened biochemical system. When these chemicals combine they enter the blood stream and go to the brain.

My hypothesis is that when brain cells fire, [this emits electromagnetic radiation] certain elements are oxidized, causing protein to dissolve. This coats brain cells and forms tangles in the brain fibers. Published research indicates that the synapse, [the space between brain cells] is littered with amyloid plaque, [clipped and or dissolved protein deposits.]

Ethan R. Signer M.D., Professor of Biology Emeritus, MIT stated in the publication from the Alzheimer Research Forum, June 8, 2000 titled, Gamma Secretase Sweepstakes: "Presenilin still in the running." Dr. Signer says, "The identity of gamma-secretase, the enzyme that frees amyloid-beta from its membrane-bound precursor, is one of the holy grails in the search for the cause of Alzheimer's disease."

I believe that Dr. Signer is correct. When my work is put to the test it may be found that gamma-secretase, the mutated enzyme and the combined food and drink chemical additives, that I have isolated will have a lot in common and may be shown as the cause of Alzheimer's dementia.

Regarding regular vanillin, we can track this further back in time and tie this in with the explorer Cortez and his return to Europe from Mexico. *The University of New South Whales, Sidney, Australia, School of Chemistry,* says, "The Aztecs used vanillin as a flavoring and it was brought to Europe by Cortez in about 1520." He brought vanilla plants with him, which contained the natural vanillin. Vanillin is the chemical that gives vanilla its flavor. Ethyl-vanillin is two or three times stronger than regular vanillin.

Huntington disease is another Neurodegenerative disease which can be traced back to the 15th century. *The Merck Manual of Medical Information, Home Edition 1997 states that,* "Huntington disease, [Huntington's chorea] is an inherited disease in which people in their midlife begin having occasional jerks and spasms and gradual loss of brain cells progressing to chorea, athetosis and mental deterioration. The gene for Huntington's disease is dominant; therefore, children of people who have this disease have a 50 percent chance of developing it."

The Harper Collins Illustrated Medical Dictionary defines Dominant as, "In genetics, a characteristic that is apparent even when the gene for it is carried by only one of a pair of homologous chromosomes."

The Harper Collins Illustrated Medical Dictionary, defines Mutagen as, "Any agent that causes a permanent, heritable change mutation in the genetic material of a cell i.e. radioactive substances, certain chemicals."

Remember Alois Alzheimer? The German Neuropathologist who diagnosed the first Alzheimer's case in 1906. Now, hold that thought while considering the following interesting information found on the web. Rhodia, one of the manufactures of vanillin [a food additive and artificial flavor] in a report titled," Extra Pure Ethyl Vanillin," *Rhodia's web site stated on April 2, 2002, that,* "The first actual description of ethyl-vanillin occurs in a German patent, registered by Schering in 1894." This would have been eleven years before doctor Alzheimer identified the disease. Can this be a coincidence?

Think about that! Alzheimer's was first diagnosed in Germany by Dr. Alois Alzheimer, a German neuropathologist.

The first patent for ethyl-vanillin was issued in Germany.

I will show in later chapters that, ethyl-vanillin is a very dangerous chemical to the mental functioning of an elderly person. I believe regular vanillin is a problem when my biochemical system weakens from aging.

My research shows that the stronger ethyl-vanillin is a much stronger oxidizer of the metals in our bodies and when combined with other chemicals in our diet is even more devastating to memory then regular vanillin.

CHAPTER THREE:
MEMORY LOSS AND
CONFUSION

I've heard it called, Alzheimer's, and I've heard it called dementia and cognitive impairment. I've also heard it called Alzheimer's disease. When it killed my mother, the doctors wrote Alzheimer's dementia on her death certificate.

When it started on me, I experienced a severe loss of memory, with a lot of confusion. I was able to reverse this condition after several years of research and testing on myself.

Regardless of what you call it, my private research reveals, my memory problems and confusion were based in element deficiency. When I replaced the deficient elements and removed certain chemicals from my diet, the memory loss and confusion went away.

My work shows methyl-eugenol and or ethyl-vanillin [artificial flavors] to be very strong oxidizers, especially in double strength form.

My work also shows propylene glycol to be a strong emulsifier and solvent. Vitamins, which are water soluble and fat soluble can be confused by strong double emulsifiers, when placed in my bodies weakened biochemical system.

When strong artificial flavors are combined with double emulsifiers, they can overpower my age weakened biochemical system.

In other words, metals are being oxidized and vitamins are being inhibited. This interferes with an enzymes ability to catalyze biochemical reactions. The oxidized metals of copper, zinc and manganese produce free radicals and interfere with the super oxide dismutase [SOD] free radical scavenger.

Metalloproteins are affected by oxidation.

Stedman's Medical Dictionary describes Metalloproteins as, "A protein containing a metal ion within its structure."

PHOTOCHEMISTRY:

In order to better understand the pathogenesis of Alzheimer's disease, I believe we must take into account the effects of photochemistry on metals. *The American Heritage Stedman's Medical Dictionary describes Photochemistry as,* "The branch of chemistry that deals with the effects of light on chemical Systems."

PHOTOEMISSION:

Merriam-Webster's Dictionary describes Photoemission as, "The release of electrons from a usu. solid material [as a metal] by means of energy supplied by incidence of radiation and especially light."

PHOTODYNAMICS:

Stedman's Medical Dictionary, describes Photodynamics as, "The science that deals with the activating effects of light on living organisms."

PHOTOLYSIS:

Stedman's Medical Dictionary describes Photolysis as, "Chemical decomposition induced by light or other radiant energy."

The **"oxidation photograph"** located on our web site at **www.zapalzheimers.com** shows the results of an experiment I conducted. I placed a new piece of aluminum foil [a metal] into a glass container, and then I added enough propylene-glycol and ethyl-vanillin to cover the aluminum foil. I then placed the glass container in the sun light for several months. [Remember, it takes years and years for the aluminum and other metals found in the amyloid plaque to form in the Alzheimer's brain.] Vanillin, when exposed to light, oxidizes and propylene-glycol acts as a solvent.

The photograph also shows the results of my experiment. After several months, the propylene-glycol and ethyl-vanillin evaporated. All of the aluminum was aggregated into a pile of aluminum oxide granules, [center photograph] leaving only the backing paper shown at the bottom of the photograph. At the beginning of the experiment, the backing paper contained a covering of aluminum and it looked like the new piece of aluminum foil shown at the top of the photograph.

If you look closely at the photograph, you can see where the propylene-glycol and ethyl-vanillin has eaten holes in the backing paper. Can there be a connection here to the Creutzfeldt-Jakob disease, [the human form of Mad Cow disease known as Bovine spongiform encephalopathy] which eats holes in the brain?

This process, no doubt, works its destruction on other elements also; say like lithium, nitrogen, fluorine, sodium, silicon, and iron. These elements are represented in the "Periodic Table of Elements" by the numbers, 3, 7, 9, 11, 14, and 26. We need these elements for good mental health. If they are inhibited through the process of oxidation, it doesn't take a rocket scientist to understand, they must be replaced or my cognition will decline. This oxidation of elements also produces unpaired electrons, commonly known as free radicals.

Yet, I do not believe aluminum was the cause of my memory deficit. Aluminum is only a small piece of the Alzheimer's puzzle.

Take a look at this! Webster's Dictionary says regarding Propylene-glycol that, "Propylene-glycol is a sweet hygroscopic viscous liquid C3H8O2 made esp. from propylene and used esp. as an antifreeze and solvent and in brake fluids." And their putting this in our foods?

I do not believe propylene glycol is a problem for the elderly until it is combined with other emulsifiers and double to triple strength ethyl vanillin or eugenol. These two are strong oxidizers.

Elderly people can be deficient in Silicon.

When I was young, the silicon in my body collected the aluminum and removed it. Now my age weakened biochemical system is allowing methyl-eugenol, ethyl-vanillin [artificial flavors] combined with propylene glycol [emulsifier and solvent that allows water and oils to mix] to inhibit the silicon in my body through the process of oxidation. [See chapter 17 titled "Conclusion" and silicon, atomic number 14.]

Methyl eugenol ethyl vanillin is known oxidizers:

Do-nut shops use propylene-glycol [emulsifier and solvent] and ethyl-vanillin [double strength oxidizer] in most of their products. Most candies, ice cream and other desserts contain methyl-eugenol, ethyl-vanillin [artificial flavors] and emulsifiers. [See Chapter 10 titled "Exposed" and chapter 11 titled "Eugenol, Vanillin and Emulsifiers."]

Twelve years ago, when I embarked on this search, it was to help my mother who was having memory problems. We suspected that it was the Alzheimer's disease, which was later confirmed. At the time, I had no idea of the unbelievable effort it would require to educate myself on the information that is written in this book, because, at the time I had no medical knowledge at all. It would have been impossible for my subconscious mind to have produced the "six numbers," that occurred in the year of 1993. Here are the facts. You decide. There are 114 known atomic elements in the Periodic Table of Elements, and over 59 of these atomic elements are found in the human body. 18 of these 59 atomic elements are necessary to sustain life.

The "six numbers" represent "six atomic elements" in the Periodic Table *and account for a full one-third of the 18 atomic elements necessary to sustain life.*

See the chart of the "Periodic Table of Elements" *at the end of chapter 18. It shows the* "six numbers" *[six atomic elements.]*

The odds of choosing the correct "six atomic elements" *from over 59 atomic elements, that may restore memory, are over 45 million to one. Think about the thousands of very bright medical researcher's worldwide researching the Alzheimer's disease.*

I want to comment here on a prescription drug. Vioxx was recently pulled from the market because of heart problems. Vioxx contained artificial flavors and emulsifiers; these are two substances that I have identified as a problem with my memory deficit and coronary artery disease by testing on myself.

In fact, I did too much testing on myself, by ingesting these combined chemicals, [artificial flavors and emulsifiers] and in August of 2004, I had to have open-heart surgery. A quadruple bypass.

I am sure Merck has not been aware of this problem with artificial flavors and emulsifiers. Someone should tell them.

After all, if Merck and others in the medical profession had been aware of eugenol, methyl-eugenol, ethyl-vanillin and vanillin combined with emulsifiers, in the elderly, would we still have as much heart disease and Alzheimer's dementia as we do?

So how does this work? We find part of the answers in *Dr. Elmer M. Cranton's* fine book on chelation therapy titled, *"Bypassing Bypass Surgery."* [Author-Please keep in mind while reading the following information that methyl-eugenol, ethyl-vanillin are oxidizers that produce free radicals.]

Dr. Cranton relates on pages 270 and 271 that, "As cholesterol becomes oxidized in the form of low-density lipoprotein [LDL] cholesterol, LDL receptor sites in the liver and elsewhere are altered causing increased hepatic synthesis of endogenous cholesterol."

Dr. Cranton further relates that, "After encountering and neutralizing a free radical, a molecule of cholesterol is oxidized as LDL cholesterol. In oxidized LDL form, cholesterol is toxic to blood vessel walls. If antioxidant protection is diminished, or if free radical production exceeds the threshold of tolerance, oxidized LDL cholesterol increases and contributes to atherosclerosis."

This is the process by which I caused major blockage in my arteries in testing on myself, by ingesting substantial quantities of methyl-eugenol and ethyl-vanillin combined with propylene glycol, which is contained in foods, mostly desserts and candies. At the time I was trying to isolate the cause of my Alzheimer's symptoms. I had no idea there was a relationship between Alzheimer's disease and atherosclerosis, which was being caused by these combined chemical additives, [artificial flavors and emulsifiers.]

Oh! By the way, I have never taken Vioxx in my life.

However, in testing on myself, over a three year period, I ingested methyl-eugenol, ethyl-vanillin, [artificial flavors] and double emulsifiers contained in desserts and candies, in abundant quantities.

Vioxx also contained artificial flavors and emulsifiers. I do not believe people in the medical field are aware of this problem with methyl-eugenol and propylene-glycol ethyl-vanillin in the elderly. This is why I am writing this book. **We need studies on this.**

To further make my point, consider the following information.

Look at the differences between Vioxx and Celebrex. Vioxx was pulled from the market place.

Why is **Vioxx causing heart problems?** Is it because **Vioxx contains artificial flavors combined with emulsifiers?**

Vioxx also contains **methyl-phenyl,** [methyl is derived from methane, which is used as a fuel, and phenyl, is a benzene derivative and close cousin to phenol.]

Why was **Celebrex causing heart problems?** Is it because **Celebrex also contains methyl-phenyl?**

Are we talking alcohol combined with phenol here? If we are, that describes ethyl-vanillin.

Why does **Celebrex lower cancer risk** and help in the **treatment of Alzheimer's disease?** Is it because it contains atomic **number 7** [nitrogen,] and atomic **number 9** [fluorine.] **Vioxx does not contain these two elements. Isn't that interesting?**

My critics will say, "Artificial flavors didn't have anything to do with my blocked arteries, let alone my memory problems."

Let's look at the facts. Four main things contribute to heart problems:

[1.] Being a heavy smoker. [I quit smoking 42 years ago.]

[2.] Having high blood pressure. [My doctor says I have the blood pressure of a 17 year old athlete, very low.]

[3.] Having high cholesterol. My cholesterol has always been normal, until I spent 3 years testing on myself ingesting the chemicals that cause Alzheimer's dementia and block arteries because metals were being oxidized. This caused an increase in my LDL cholesterol [low density lipoprotein.]

[4.] Being a heavy drinker. [I doubt I average 2 drinks a week.]

Since I have never consumed a lot of bad fats in my diet, the only thing left to consider are the chemicals I ingested. These are contained in desserts, like in candies, ice cream, pastries [artificial flavors.]

In the following chapters I will share with you the things I have found out through the process of an elimination diet, over a three year testing period on myself. This process of an elimination diet, revealed to me what caused my memory deficit. As you might imagine, it was complicated.

Discuss this information with your doctor. He or she is the doctor in charge of your health care. If you feel my information has merit, and your doctor rejects it, try a different doctor.

Remember you are the one who is dealing daily with the loved one who has all these problems, not the doctor.

If you do not take matters into your own hands, then next year may be harder than the past year. A restored memory could make life fun again.

This dementia has been on the books over 100 years. However, I believe senility has existed much longer then that. Three combined substances in food and drink, alcohol, eugenol and emulsifiers in their original form, can be dated back to China, 2000 BC.

These three combined substances would have been alcohol [spirits], eugenol [clove oil or other spices] and emulsifiers [eggs.] These three combined substances when placed in an aged persons body, in my opinion, would have caused dementia and memory problems because of a weakened biochemical system.

As long as we are talking about China, **Parkinson's disease** is one thing to consider.

Worldwide, there are 4 million cases of Parkinson's disease. Why, are almost 50% of the worldwide cases of Parkinson's in China? I believe it has to do with the same things that are involved in Alzheimer's disease, namely, eugenol, alcohol, and emulsifiers. **Think about the orient and spices [which contain eugenol.]**

In 1999, Alzheimer's disease killed my mother. Doctor's did not know what caused the Alzheimer's disease or how to reverse it. Several years before Mother died, I became aware of the 6 numbers, but I did not understand them. It took me years to figure it out. Too late to help Mother, I'm sorry to say. These 6 numbers became the formula that reversed my memory deficit.

I understand this is next to impossible to believe. If someone told me this story, I would also be very skeptical. I have a suggestion, why don't we use science to evaluate the six numbers? I think when you see that the 6 numbers [six elements] are definitely involved in Alzheimer's dementia you will come to the proper conclusion.

I am using these numbers [elements] successfully to treat myself today. My brain cells are free of the deadly beta amyloid plaque. You see, about the time of my mother's death, this disease came after me. Alzheimer's had started doing to my mind the same things it did to my mother's, before it eventually killed her. Although I really wanted to help my mother early on, I knew nothing about where to start looking. I only knew they were finding aluminum particles in Alzheimer's brains. I could make nothing of this, except, I knew aluminum was an electrical conductor. Only about 60 % as efficient as copper. This was of no help.

When this disease started on me, I knew if I did not want to end up like Mom, I had only one chance, figure it out or else now, I had something to work with. I could use my body as a testing laboratory. During the next three years, using a process of elimination diet I was able to isolate what I believe was the cause of my Alzheimer's symptoms. The same symptoms my mother had. Then by ingesting more food then normal which contained these combined chemical additives, I was able to do in-depth testing on myself that produced advanced Alzheimer's symptoms.

During this testing period on myself, I have heard common words spoken and had to think hard to understand their meanings. I heard sentences spoken, and to this day, I do not know what was said. Once during a testing period on myself, I came to an intersection while driving, one that I know well. This time I recognized nothing and turned the wrong way. It was extreme confusion and at times I was unable to perform normal chores. I have stood in front of a mirror in the morning and could not remember why I was there. I have rubbed toothpaste on my face instead of shaving lotion, then thought, what did I do that for.

Numbers are a big problem also. When my mind was confused, it was as if a wall had gone up. It was as if my mind was out of gear. It was hard to think progressively. One minute I was trying to focus on something and a couple minutes later the whole thought was gone. If I tried to reclaim it, then, it became even more confusing. I remember one night when I was in a testing period on myself; it took me 20 minutes to set the alarm clock. I kept getting confused between alarm time and current time.

When a person has Alzheimer's, numbers are a huge problem especially the balancing of a check book. I think the problems with numbers may be an early indicator of the onset of Alzheimer's. Once during testing on myself, I woke up looked at the clock, read it wrong, got dressed and drove to the corner. The vehicle clock said 1:00 a.m. my wristwatch said 1:00 a.m. so I went back to bed. I noticed other things also like reaching for the heater or radio switches, instead of turning it on, I turned it off. I caught myself doing this a lot, turning switches the wrong way. This has never been a problem for me. In the past, it was always automatic without even thinking about it.

Being in this state of mind was like a nightmare, best described as descending into the abyss. It was very scary. I did not want to go back in there anymore.

I remember once, when I had caused advanced Alzheimer's symptoms by testing on myself, and I needed to go across town to a location near the Astrodome. In my minds eye, I could see where I wanted to go, [the location] I had one problem; I couldn't get it in my mind just what roads I needed to take to get there. So I stayed home. "In my 35 years in Houston, Texas, I have driven over 300,000 miles on Houston streets, and I know the city like the back of my hand."

I remember the expressions on my poor Mothers face when she was confused and frustrated. I never really knew what it was like, until I experienced it myself. After experiencing the thing about words and sentences, I realized why. When I talked to Mother in the later stages of her Alzheimer's, she would only stare at me. If she tried to talk, we could not understand her. She had lost the ability to form and understand words.

Love must be the strongest emotion we have. Once when I told my mother, "I love you," although she could not speak other words, she managed to murmur the almost understandable words, "I love you too."

I have thought time after time how I prayed for a way to help my mother, but I did not understand the *"six numbers."* The element replacement therapy [using the 6 elements] restored my normal cognition and my memory. I will reveal in a later chapter more details.

I would like to take this opportunity to present a challenge to all neuroscientists anywhere on this planet. Take this information into your laboratories and put it to the test.

CHAPTER FOUR:
THE PUZZLE

This work has been like a giant puzzle, but,

Instead of the pieces having shapes, pictures, and colors to identify how everything fits into the big picture, the pieces of this puzzle have been words and sentences. Mostly of which I did not know their definitions, and also had trouble pronouncing them.

Seven years ago, I did not know how to use a computer, or how to use it for research. Now, I can within minutes, download enormous amounts of information on any subject I am interested in. This has been a great help for me, because of my curious mind. In the past I had to drive to the downtown library, where I would spend all day Saturday and half of Sundays, researching things I was interested in.

Examining another piece of the puzzle. The Blood Brain Barrier [BBB.]

Regarding the BBB the web site, http://faculty.washington.edu/chudler/bbb.html *says,* "Over 100 years ago, it was discovered, that if blue dye was injected into the blood stream of an animal, that tissues of the whole body EXCEPT the brain and spinal cord would turn blue. To explain this, scientists thought that a Blood Brain-Barrier [BBB] which prevents materials from the blood from entering the brain existed. More recently, scientists have discovered much more about the structure and function of the BBB." *Continuing on the web site says,*

"The BBB is semi-permeable; that is it allows some materials to cross, but prevents others from crossing."

The Harper Collins Illustrated Medical Dictionary, states, "The Blood Brain Barrier [BBB] the tight junction between endothelial cells of the capillary walls that normally permits only a limited exchange between bloods in the capillaries, on the one hand and cerebrospinal fluid and extracellular fluid in the brain on the other."

So, what are the things that can open the BBB that would allow a toxic compound to enter?

The web site, http://faculty.washington.edu/chudler/bbb.html,

Says, "There are seven ways this can occur." The site defines them as:

1. "Hypertension   [high blood pressure.]
2. Trauma, brain injury, or... inflammation.
3. Infection.
4. Radiation.
5. Not a fully developed BBB as in a newborn.
6. Microwaves.
7. A high concentration of a substance in the blood."

Let's concentrate on one of the ways to open the BBB. "Inflammation," Non-steroidal anti-inflammatory drugs [Nsaid's] is helping in the treatment of Alzheimer's disease, by reducing inflammation. According to statistics, about 50% of the patients in the early stages of dementia have found the symptoms reduced when using Nsaid's. This is not a cure and there can be side effects. Is it possible, when inflammation is reduced, the BBB may go back up and may stop the toxic proteins and mutated enzymes from entering the brain?

Another piece of the puzzle:

Joe Graedon and Teresa Graedon, related in their column, in the Houston Chronicle, Friday, Nov. 2, 2001 that, "At least four readers have written in and claimed that relatives, husbands, wives, mothers and fathers who suffered with Alzheimer's, had became completely lucid when given narcotic pain relievers, the mental cognitive impairment disappeared. They were like their old self's again, until the medication wore off, then the problems with dementia returned."

So what are we to make of this?

Well, re: pain killers, *The Mosby Medical Encyclopedia Revised Edition, states that,* "Pain, is a basic symptom of inflammation."

The inflammation is stopped and with what results? The BBB may be closed again, and in my opinion, the combined chemical additives in food and drink that may be rendering the proteins and enzymes toxic, are possibly being blocked from entering the brain.

In the case of the Nsaid's, some contain sodium.

Sodium [Na] contains 11 protons in its nucleus and is atomic number 11, in the Periodic Table.

Sodium is extremely reactive chemically.

So is sodium important in the brain?

Judge for yourself. *The Funk & Wagnalls Atlas of the Body,* says, "Sodium [Na] and its counterpart potassium [k] are two of the most abundantly occurring elements in nature. The brain will not function without electrically charged sodium ions" *The Atlas continues on to say,* "Sodium's workmate potassium also has electrically charged ions. Nerve impulse conduction uses the movement of the electrically charged ions across the nerve cell membrane. When a nerve cell is polarized or at rest, there are more positive charged potassium [k +] ions, than positive charged sodium [Na +] ions, inside the cell. There is an opposite ratio outside the cell."

Describing this further, the Atlas says, "Sodium [Na +] ions are kept out of the cell by an energy consuming pump mechanism," [Author- the sodium-potassium pump.] "This maintains a negative charge inside the cell, and a positive charge outside the cell. When a thought impulse travels along the nerve, sodium ions flood into the cell and make the inside of the nerve cell positive, with respect to the outside of the cell. When this happens, the cell is excited, and referred to as depolarized. This condition is called an action potential. Action potentials move rapidly from one cell to another." *The Atlas says,* "The waves of alteration in a molecular structure, and inflow and outflow of ions, to and from nerve cells, constitute a nerve impulse."

Explaining the process further the Atlas says, "After a nerve cell has been depolarized, it will revert to a polarized state. However, until the molecules and ions have been rearranged it is not excitable, and will not conduct impulses, and is referred to as refractory [unmanageable.]" *The Atlas says,* "Some thought impulses travel at speeds up to 300 feet per second. Medical information states that our bodies contain more than 10,000 million nerve cells that make up our nervous system."

The Funk and Wagnalls Atlas of the Body is a very well written and informative book.

Let's think about that, "300 feet per second." That means a thought impulse in a six foot man or woman could travel from head to toe 50 times in one second. That's what I call, "rapid communication."

A lack of sodium [Na +] ions, atomic number 11 in the Periodic Table of Elements, certainly would cause problems in the memory process.

So how does this work? A thought comes to mind. If the sodium needs replacing, then something is wrong with the sodium that needs to be replaced. Are these combined chemicals oxidizing the sodium, altering the polarity of the sodium, rendering it electrically static, [blocking its electrical charge?] This may explain the presence of dementia with amyloid plaque, and dementia when there is no amyloid plaque. As we will see in Gene's case, in Chapter 5 titled, *"Fitting Key Pieces Together."* Gene was a childhood friend who passed away with memory impairment.

Somewhere in this malfunction lies the answer to the build up of amyloid plaque [dissolved protein] in the synaptic cleft [the space between nerve cells.] A breakdown of electrical function, between nerve cells, [a space that has to be crossed electrically, in order for memory and thought processes to function,] could result in accelerated cognitive impairment.

CHAPTER FIVE:
FITTING KEY PIECES TOGETHER

Follow along with me. See how I try to fit together more pieces of words and sentences which, I hope will shed some light on how these combined chemical food and drink additives may be causing this destructive disease called, Alzheimer's dementia. That's when my body will no longer process these chemicals without the memory problems. After I search out these pieces of information, I must look up their definitions. More times than not after the time and trouble involved, some pieces of information must be discarded if they have no merit.

However, two of the following pieces look promising, Hydergine and Thiamine. Before examining these let me say, these two pieces of the puzzle came from Gene, a childhood friend who passed away June 17, 2001, in Miami, Florida. These two medications were prescribed for Gene on July 13, 1998, at the nursing home where he was admitted on July 6, 1998. Gene was my age, he had two older brothers, Jamer in the middle and Dee was the oldest.

Dee also passed away recently. His death was caused by Amyotropic Lateral Sclerosis [ALS] or commonly known as Lou Gehrig's disease. [A Neurodegenerative disease.]

Growing up in post World War II, Miami, Florida, these three brothers lived a couple blocks up the street from me. Their home was right on the banks of a canal. An extension of Miami's little river canal.

When we were not in school, we were swimming in that canal. What great childhood memories.

I asked Jamer to send me copies of Gene's medical papers and autopsy reports. I wanted to peer over the doctor's shoulders to see what I might perceive. How it might tie in with my research into Alzheimer's dementia. Follow along with me to see what we might learn from this.

Gene was diagnosed with Alzheimer's on July 17, 1998. Then after another diagnosis on June 10, 2001, Alzheimer's was confirmed a second time.

After Gene's death, June 16, 2001, *an autopsy clinical diagnosis states the chief disease as ALS. Then on June 17, 2001 the neuropathology report describes,* possible Parkinson's disease. [A different diagnosis.] In the final analysis, the report stated "Cause of death, unknown." I have tremendous respect for people with small "ego's," who are not afraid to say, "We don't know." Whether they are medical professionals or wheat farmers, they are being honest.

I examined Gene's medical records further and I saw three things that were striking, and needed to be considered. First, when Gene was admitted to the nursing home July 6, 1998, *the report stated,* "He was given double portions of regular diet because of his poor nutrition." Nutrition is a word that should be gold plated for later recognition. *The report stated,* "He slept well and his appetite was good." This statement was an oxymoron. "He ate well and he was losing weight." *The autopsy report stated,* "The body is that of an under nourished white man. The body appears to be older than the stage age of 66 years. The body weighs approx. 85 pounds." Good grief, almost 70 pounds had disappeared since Gene became ill with this disease.

Two new "word pieces" of this puzzle we are trying to piece together are malabsorption and its first cousin, malnutrition.

Regarding malabsorption and malnutrition, the Mayo Clinic Family Health Book, Second Edition, states, "If the process of digestion is to go smoothly, the nutrients contained in the food you eat must be broken down [digested] into molecules that can be absorbed into your bloodstream. Sometimes, for various reasons, these nutrients are not completely digested or their absorption is impaired. When this occurs, vital nutrients that should be used by your body instead are eliminated in the stool. The result of this malabsorption can be malnutrition."

Wow! The golden word "Nutrition." My hypothesis is that, "Nutrients are not being absorbed properly into the blood stream from the small intestine." This is so important that I think I will say it again, "Nutrients are not being absorbed properly into the blood stream, from the small intestine."

The doctors were trying to decide which one of the deadly neurological diseases took Gene's life, and they could not decide. The first cousin malnutrition get's my vote. Gene's body could not get enough nutrition to sustain life. Which organ shut down is irrelevant. Organs also need nutrition to sustain life. This situation is evident in almost any Alzheimer's care facility, people just waste away.

Remember, in chapter 3 that, eighteen of over fifty-nine atomic elements found in the human body are necessary to sustain life. Six of those eighteen atomic elements are involved in Alzheimer's dementia. Think about that, 18 atomic elements out of over 59 atomic elements found in the human body which are necessary to maintain life, a full one third of the 18 atomic elements [six numbers] are definitely involved in Alzheimer's. Expanding on this even further, consider the odds of choosing the correct 6 numbers ["six atomic elements"] out of the 114 atomic elements. See odds calculator at the end of this chapter.

How many people who's loved ones lives, have been touched by Alzheimer's disease, do you think have prayed for a miracle?

Ok, remember the two word pieces of this neuro puzzle, Hydergine and Thiamine, the prescribed medications for Gene. *The Mosby Medical Encyclopedia, Revised Edition, defines Hydergine as,* "A Trademark for a drug to treat peripheral vein disease." Hydergine is recommended for early and middle stages of Alzheimer's, although it will not reverse or stop this disease. Because of Gene's poor nutrition, the doctors were trying to increase the volume of blood to the brain.

The Merck Manual of Medical Information, Home Edition states that, "Thiamine is of the B complex vitamin group. Thiamine joins with pyruvic acid to form a coenzyme necessary for the breakdown of carbohydrates into glucose." So it is evident the doctors were trying to increase nutrition and strengthen the nervous system.

The Mosby Medical Encyclopedia, Revised Edition, states that, "A lack of thiamine affects chiefly the nervous system, the circulation, the stomach and intestines."

The Mosby Medical Encyclopedia, describes Pyruvic acid as, "A compound formed by processing glucose where there is oxygen."

The Merck Manual of Medical Information states, "Absence of Pyruvate carboxylase an enzyme interferes with or blocks the production of glucose in the body."

I think the combined chemical additives in food and drink that Gene's immune and biochemical defense system could no longer counter, disarmed the pyruvic acid, thereby rendering the thiamine [vitamin B-1] ineffective.

Mitochondria produce ATP:

The Mosby Medical Encyclopedia, defines Mitochondria as, "A small, thread like organ within the cytoplasm of a cell that controls cell life and breathing. Mitochondria are the main source of cell energy." Mitochondria convert carbohydrates, fats and protein into adenosine triphosphate [ATP.] This supplies the energy to our cells. When our bodies can no longer breakdown carbohydrates properly, how can the body extract nutrition from the food?

These following words from *Trace Mineral Research, tells the whole story.* "Trace minerals through biochemical communication; send "Nutrients" to areas of the body that are most in need of help."

There is that word again, "Nutrition."

My findings are that combined chemicals in our food and drink are inhibiting certain "trace elements." I believe this is caused by a degeneration of an age related, weakened immune and biochemical defense system. In addition, in my opinion, a person with Alzheimer's, who continues to eat food and drink containing these combined chemicals, may find their mental condition, continuing to deteriorate because the *"six elements"* are being inhibited. On the other hand, if a person is not having memory problems these combined chemical food and drink additives may not be a problem, until the person enters old age.

Vitamin E, also called Tocopherol, was also prescribed for Gene. Vitamin E is an excellent antioxidant. It works to remove free radicals that are responsible for the degeneration of brain cells.

Vitamin E can inhibit iron [atomic number 26] in the body.

Vitamin C tends to mobilize the bodies iron store, which is why I use vitamin E combined with vitamin C.

Gene was also given folic acid. Folic acid is of the B complex and needed for cell growth. Folic acid functions with vitamin B-12 and vitamin C in the breakdown of protein, and in making hemoglobin. It also increases the appetite and plays a role in the production of hydrochloric acid in the stomach.

Re: Homocysteine

Dr. David Snowdon's well-known Kentucky Nun's study has shown that, "Low levels of Vitamin B-6, B-12 and folic acid in the blood can cause methionine [an essential protein building block] to convert into a poison called homocysteine. Studies show that a high level of homocysteine, in the blood can put a person at risk for Alzheimer's disease." More information on this can be found in Dr. David A. Snowdon's book titled, "Aging With Grace."

Maybe, all that Gene's doctor's had to do was replace the "six elements" on a regular basis that were being disarmed by combined chemicals in his food and drink. In my opinion, his body could not process the combined chemicals anymore because of his age-weakened immune and biochemical defense system. Were the trace elements in his body being oxidized by methyl-eugenol, ethyl-vanillin, [oxidizers] and propylene-glycol [emulsifier and solvent] from the food and drink he was ingesting, creating mutated enzymes?

Alzheimer's disease is a complicated process.

Although Gene and I both ate these combined chemical additives all our lives in our food and drink, we remained healthy until we reached 50 to 65 years of age. When our bodies get older, the normal processing of the combined chemicals in our food and drink slow down, then cognitive impairment and other problems may set in.

When I replace the *"six elements"* in my body, on a continual basis, my mind is as sharp as ever. When I go without replacing these *"six elements,"* on a regular basis, the cognitive impairment starts to increase and multiplies the confusion and other symptoms. The very things my mother described.

Because of Gene's Alzheimer's symptoms, on July 13, 1998, doctors prescribed Aricept for the dementia. Aricept is an inhibitor of the cholinesterase that breaks down and strips choline from the acetylcholine neurotransmitter. Blocking this process makes more choline available for use. But this did not stop Gene's Alzheimer's disease. *In the neurological assessment on June 10, 2001, the report states,* "The patient is awake and non-communicative." Seven days later Gene passed away.

Reading further in the autopsy report we find information that is unsuspected. One would think with two diagnosis of Alzheimer's, there would be definite markings in the brain. *The report states,* "Neither lewy bodies [senile plaques] nor neurofibrillary tangles [tau,] are seen. The spinal cord appears normal." What this tells me is, although Gene was diagnosed twice with Alzheimer's disease, the doctors could not find any beta amyloid plaque during the post mortem autopsy of his brain.

In Dr. John Medina's book, titled, "What you need to know about Alzheimer's," he states, "Plaques are spherelike structures, existing just outside nerve cells called senile plaques by Dr. Alzheimer. They are surrounded by degenerating axon terminals and dendrite branches."

Dr. Medina defines tangles [tau] as, "Abnormal structures, found inside the nerve cells of Alzheimer's patients. They are highly ordered bundles of molecules that can kill the nerve cells in which they reside."

No wonder the hombres down at the "Neuro Sweat Shop" are in such a dither trying to sort this out.

Wait a minute! Common logic is trying to kick in. Let's see! There is dementia and cognitive impairment and loss of synaptic transmission in the presence of amyloid plaque and tau tangles. In Gene's case he had these same symptoms but there were no markings of amyloid plaques or tau tangles?

Logic dictates this question, are there two culprits at work here? One is producing toxic protein, killing brain cells near the toxic plaques and causing tau tangles to form in brain fibers, shutting down memory. The other culprit is also shutting down memory but leaves no visible evidence. A thought comes to mind here, I have read that the energy level in the brain of Alzheimer's patients is less than in a normal brain.

This brings to mind another piece of the *"word puzzle,"* that bounced around in my brain, from neuron to neuron for six or eight months. Mitochondria, this "dynamic dynamo" provides the energy used by the cells of our body.

Imagine this, my cell phone battery was low, and I couldn't communicate. Even with web access I could not access memory. Hmmm.....

As long as we are on the subject of energy, here is more information regarding the mitochondria. *The Harper Collins Illustrated Medical Dictionary, describes the mitochondria as,* "One of numerous compartmentalized, self reproducing organelles present in the cytoplasm of most cells. It has its own DNA and is responsible for generating usable energy by the formation of adenosine triphosphate [ATP.] The average cell contains several hundred mitochondria." This is an excellent book and very well written.

Another thought recalled. Researchers examining the plaque and debris in Alzheimer's brains, found deposits of sugars and phosphates. Two more "word pieces" of this puzzle. Set them aside for a moment. Remember mitochondria convert carbohydrates, fats and protein into adenosine triphosphate. ATP is composed of a base [adenosine], a sugar [ribose], and three phosphate groups. Ding-dong! Did I hear a bell go off? Sugars and phosphates found in plaques!

Can these combined chemicals in food and drinks... wait, let's back up. I know positively they are responsible. I just spent 3 years isolating them as the cause of my Alzheimer's symptoms, just exactly like Mother's symptoms. The only thing to figure out is how they are doing it. Neuroscientists call this, "the mechanism of action."

As an impulse or message is transmitted between brain cells an electrical charge is emitted as charged sodium ions [Na+] flood into the cell to displace the potassium ions [K+] and depolarize the cell. When this occurs, an electro-magnetic-field [Emf] is produced. This may be one "mechanism of action."

Tryptophan is another piece of the *"word puzzle,"* a real jewel. Tryptophan [Trp] is an amino acid. Tryptophan is the precursor of the neurotransmitter serotonin. Serotonin is an organic compound also called 5- hydroxytryptamine. *Stedman's Medical Dictionary, describes Serotonin as,* "Active in vasoconstriction, transmission of impulses between nerve cells and regulation of cyclic body processes."

The Mosby Medical Encyclopedia, defines vasoconstriction as, "A narrowing of any blood vessel, especially the arterioles and the veins in the blood reservoirs of the skin and the abdominal viscera." *Mosby goes on to describe the Viscera as,* "The internal organs within the body, mainly the stomach and intestines." Blood gives nutrients and oxygen to the cells and collects waste from the cells.

Question? If a person is at risk for Alzheimer's, [his or her body may no longer process these combined chemical additives,] where does this food and drink containing these artificial flavors and emulsifiers go when they are ingested? Of course, into the stomach and on to the small intestine.

Nutrition has to start in the stomach and small intestine, right?

My findings are, when my body can no longer process these three combined chemicals, they form a toxin or free radicals that may alter tryptophan, and serotonin. The amino acid tryptophan, [Trp] is also the basis for niacin, another *"word piece"* of this puzzle. Niacin is also of the B complex group of vitamins. Niacin [vitamin B-3] acts in the breakdown and use of all major foods. *The Mosby Medical Encyclopedia Revised Edition, refers to Niacin as,* "Necessary for the normal working of the stomach and intestinal tract. Niacin is a white crystal like vitamin of the B complex group that dissolves in water."

Suppose water was not 100% water. It is obvious that niacin could not completely perform the function of breaking down our food. More on this later, concerning emulsifiers in Chapter 11 titled *"Eugenol, Vanillin and Emulsifiers."*

Toxic chemical additives effecting tryptophan, serotonin and niacin certainly could have a bearing on the bodies non-absorption of nutrients. Remember malabsorption and malnutrition?

"Think Nutrition."

The Mosby Medical Encyclopedia, defines Schizophrenia as, "Anyone of a large group of mental disorders in which the patient loses touch with reality and can no longer think, talk or act normally."

This is really striking a cord here. My mother had a good sense of humor. May God bless you Mom. I remember a couple of years before Mom passed away, a time when she was still able to communicate and seemed to walk continuously, but she was having trouble differentiating between reality and fiction. One night we were sitting outside and Mom was inside watching TV. She came running out telling us "There was something wrong because the police were here." The police were on the television!

In testing on myself, I have experienced just a touch of this a couple of times. It was weird; it was as if I did not have the presence of mind to comprehend fully the situation. I think it goes along with not being aware of the proper use of clothing or probably other things in their proper functional setting concerning Alzheimer's.

Here again, I see how combined chemicals in my diet that my body will no longer process, may effect and alter amino acids, enzymes and neurotransmitters. We can carry this further and ask are these combined chemicals also altering other neurotransmitters like Parkinson's dopamine, by affecting the amino acid tyrosine needed to produce dopamine?

How about the many other neurotransmitters involved in multiple neurodegenerative diseases. One example is Huntington's disease. My sister Phyllis lost her husband, Denzel [Dizzy] Jones, to this terrible disease. Diz was my best friend for years, we raced stock cars together, flew airplanes together and built houses together. This horrible disease not only killed him, it killed his Mother, all his brothers and sisters and his oldest daughter Sandra, my niece. May they all rest in peace.

Amyotrophic Lateral Sclerosis [ALS] is another neurodegenerative disease that has afflicted my family. ALS took the life of Dee, the oldest of the three brothers, my childhood friends in Miami. Dee was married to my cousin Shirley. Gene was his youngest brother.

There are several of these neurodegenerative diseases. Is it possible when the immune system weakens, these combined chemical food and drink additives turn toxic and may play a role in some of these other diseases?

It seems obvious that our Creator has received more than 12 million prayers worldwide regarding dementia and Alzheimer's disease.

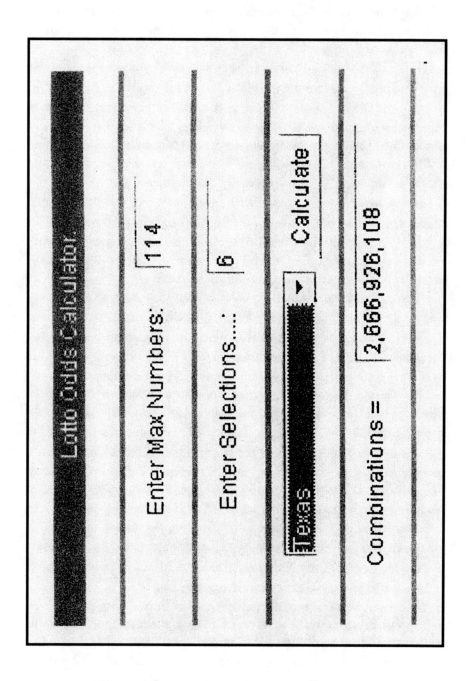

Lotto Odds Calculator

Enter Max Numbers: 114

Enter Selections....: 6

Texas ▶

Calculate

Combinations = 2,666,926,108

38

CHAPTER SIX:
ION-INTERACTION

Ion-interaction is...
utilizing enzymes, vitamins and minerals,
or is it...
"Non ion-interaction ala the emulsifier?"

Commenting on **biochemical reactions,** *Degussa Health and Nutrition Facts, says,* "Most of them are supported by biological catalysts known as enzymes. A catalyst is a substance that increases the specificity and the rate of a reaction without being changed itself.

Enzymes are proteins and the information for their biosynthesis is encoded in the DNA. In addition, many enzymes contain cofactors that increase the enzymes ability to catalyze a reaction." *Degussa goes on to say,* "Cofactors can be metal ions or organic molecules known as coenzymes." [Author-think about metal chelation and inhibited oxidized metals.] *Degussa, further relates that,* "Many cofactors of enzymes are derived from vitamins and minerals essential nutrients that cannot be synthesized by humans and mammals and therefore have to be taken in the diet." [Author- think emulsifier and artificial flavor compromised vitamins and minerals.] *Degussa, goes on to say, that,* "The human body contains an estimated number of 50,000 different enzymes."

So, you can see from the above information, that, compromised metals, vitamins and minerals would interfere with the enzymes ability to catalyze biochemical reactions.

Is this why we have Cox 2 inhibitors on the market, because, cyclooxygenase [master enzymes] are mutated? Are the oxidizers, methyl-eugenol and ethyl-vanillin the source of these mutated enzymes?

An article in the newspaper Houston Chronicle, USA, titled, "Pump up the Vitamin Volume," says, "There are more than 40 vitamin and minerals essential to the body that it cannot manufacture." *The study conducted by Dr. Robert Fletcher and Dr. Kathleen Fairfield, both of Harvard Medical School, found that,* "Low levels of folic acid and vitamins B-6 and B-12, are a risk factor for heart disease, neural tube defects and some cancers." *They report that,* "Inadequate levels of vitamin D contribute to osteoporosis and fractures. Sub-optimal amounts of the anti-oxidant vitamins A, E and C may increase the risk of cancer and heart disease." *The article says,* "Vitamins are vital to mental alertness, and they spur on chemical reactions."

Spur on chemical reactions?
Hold that thought.

Mitochondrian, in the cells of our body convert carbohydrates, proteins and fats into adenosine triphosphate [ATP]. This energy conversion from foods is accomplished through a process called cellular respiration. *Stedman's Medical Dictionary describes "Cellular Respiration," as,* "The series of metabolic processes by which living cells produce energy through the oxidation of organic substances."

I am working towards a point here!

In the book titled, "Anatomy & Physiology for Dummies," it says, "The reactions that convert fuel to usable energy include glycolysis, the Krebs cycle, and oxidative phosphorylation." *The book continues on to say,* "Altogether, these reactions are referred to as cellular respiration."

Remember in Chapter five, titled,

"Fitting Key Pieces Together," *I mentioned that the energy level in the Alzheimer's brain had been reported as lower than in a normal brain.*

Emulsifiers:

Enter the emulsifier that allows water and oils to mix. Are these water soluble and fat-soluble vitamins confused? Think about vitamins and minerals, and their effect on ionic interactions within our body.

Vitamins are designed to be either water soluble or fat-soluble. No doubt, there is a reason to divide them.

Vitamins A, D, E and K, are stored in body fat and are called fat-soluble vitamins. The B-vitamins and vitamin-C are water-soluble.

The emulsifiers allow water and oils to mix. Does this allow vitamins to go where they were not intended to go, when our bodies age and our immune system and biochemical system weakens?

One example is thiamine [water soluble vitamin B-1.] Do the emulsifiers allow thiamine to be stored in body fat? If so, how can it be available to perform the required biochemical functions?

In Chapter five titled *"Fitting Key Pieces Together,"* we saw that thiamine [B-1] joins with pyruvic acid to form a co-enzyme necessary for the breakdown of carbohydrates into glucose. A lack of thiamine affects chiefly the nervous system, [like neurons in the brain] the circulation, the stomach and the intestines.

Do emulsifiers allow fat-soluble vitamins like Vitamin-E, an important anti-oxidant, to mix with water-soluble vitamins and then be flushed out of the body in urine? If this were the case, there would be less help in removing free radicals from our bodies. Think about it!

The Mosby Medical Encyclopedia, reports the following information regarding vitamin functions, "Folic acid, also called folacin or vitamin B-9 is needed for cell growth and reproduction. *Mosby says,* "It functions with B-12 and vitamin-C in the breakdown of proteins and in the making of hemoglobin." *The Mosby Medical Encyclopedia, further says,* "Folic acid increases the appetite and causes the making of hydrochloric acid in the stomach."

Folic acid is a B vitamin and is water soluble. Does mixing an emulsifier with this water soluble B-vitamin now allow it to be stored in body fat, thereby making it unavailable for cell growth and reproduction? Does mixing folic acid, B-12 and Vitamin-C with an emulsifier, mean they may be unavailable when needed for breaking down proteins and making hemoglobin because, possibly they are being stored in body fat instead? As an example, can the function of "electron transport" be inhibited, because an emulsifier is altering the water or fat-soluble vitamins?

Here is the point.

If the vitamins and minerals are not spurring on chemical reactions, to properly breakdown carbohydrates, proteins and fats into the cell energy, adenosine triphosphate [ATP] that powers cells, **would not the Alzheimer's brain wind up with less energy to function with?** To back this point up, consider what *"Degussa Health and Nutrition," says, regarding the speed of properly catalyzed biochemical reactions,* "Reactions that are catalyzed by enzymes can be up to one trillion times faster than the corresponding reaction without catalyst." **Think cognitive impairment. Better yet, think Alzheimer's disease.**

Regarding ion-interaction, Trace Minerals Research says, "The key players in creating the electric energy within our body are structures called ions. An ion is an atom or group of atoms carrying an electric charge by virtue of having gained or lost one or more valence electrons. Valence electrons are those electrons in the outer ring of electrons orbiting the nucleus of an atom." *Trace Minerals Research also says,* "Minerals in ionic form have unique properties that distinguish them from each other and allow them to freely take part in biochemical communication throughout the body. These communications help nutrients move to those areas of the body that are in most need of their help."

Regarding vitamins and minerals, the MayoClinic.Com web site, says, "Vitamins and minerals are substances your body needs in small amounts for normal growth, function and health." *Continuing on, the site says,* "Together, vitamins and minerals are called micronutrients. Your body can't make most micronutrients, so you must get them from the foods you eat, or in some cases, from trace mineral and vitamin supplements."

For more information on vitamins and minerals, visit our web site at www.zapalzheimers.com.

CHAPTER SEVEN:
AMINO ACIDS NEUROTRANSMITTERS AND MODULATION

The Mosby Medical Encyclopedia, defines the Neurotransmitter as, "Any chemical that changes or results in the sending of nerve signals across spaces [synapses] separating nerve fibers." *Mosby also relates that,* "The body uses many neurotransmitters. These neurotransmitters are contained in sack like containers at the axon [nerve body] ends or knobs of the cell."

Thinking is impaired without neurotransmitters:

Dr. C. Kutscher relates online the following educational information titled, "Notes on Chapter 4, Carlson Psychopharmacology," Dr. Kutscher says,

"The neurotransmitter is a chemical which because of its three-dimensional structure will fit precisely into a receptor site on the neuron. The transmitter is called a ligand and is analogous to a key. The receptor site is analogous to a lock. When the ligand sits on the receptor site, it modifies the postsynaptic neuron in some way. Usually it hyperpolarizes it and makes a nerve impulse more difficult to fire or it depolarizes it slightly and makes that neuron easier to fire." *Dr. Kutscher says,* "If hyperpolarization occurs the postsynaptic membrane becomes more difficult to fire and we call the event an inhibitory postsynaptic potential [IPSP.] If a slight depolarization occurs, the cell becomes easier to fire and we call the event an excitatory postsynaptic event [EPSP.]"

Amino acids and neurotransmitters:

The Mosby Medical Encyclopedia, Revised Edition, describes the amino acid as, "An organic compound necessary for forming peptides, a piece of protein, and proteins. Digestion releases the individual amino acids from food. Amino acids are the basic structures of neurotransmitters. These amino acids are also the building blocks of proteins."

The combined chemical additives I have isolated in a process of elimination diet, methyl-eugenol, ethyl-vanillin [artificial flavors] and emulsifiers may be unbalancing the electron transport system, interfering with cell energy, and the mitochondrian production of adenosine triphosphate [ATP.] Could this explain, low energy levels in Alzheimer's patients brains? When my body no longer will process the combined chemical additives, in food and drink, do the *"six elements"* become disarmed, and do I become at risk for Alzheimer's dementia? Do amino acids then become mutated and combined with the proteins, do they disrupt the normal functioning of the neurotransmitters, and cause an over supply or under supply [the modulation if you will] in their production efforts?

Sodium [atomic number 11] is moved from the intestine to the bodies cells by a special transporter protein, and then, by an energy dependent adenosine triphosphate [ATP] mechanism. Iron [atomic number 26] is moved into the blood from the intestine, by a transporter protein named transferrin.

Methyl-eugenol, ethyl-vanillin [artificial flavors] combined with emulsifiers, may be interfering with sodium and iron transporter proteins, made from altered amino acids. Mitochondria production of ATP from carbohydrates, fats and protein contain these combined chemical additives. They may be causing a transport problem for sodium, in the secondary step of transportation of sodium.

The amino acids need nitrogen, [atomic number 7] for nitrogen balance. If the amino acids are altered by these combined chemicals and unable to deliver nitrogen, then isn't the stage set for negative nitrogen balance? *The Mosby Medical Encyclopedia, states that,* "Negative nitrogen balance occurs when more nitrogen is released than is taken in, causing the waste or destruction of tissue." When tissue is destroyed, inflammation shows up. Non-steriodal anti-inflammatory drugs

[Nsaid's] are used as a method to treat inflammation in Alzheimer's disease.

When I think of the control mechanisms of the cell, the nucleus containing the deoxyribonucleic acid [DNA,] or in the cytoplasm, especially the areas transcripting protein from ribonucleic acid [RNA,] is it possible these toxins may be responsible for over production of Ab1 – 42 peptide, the toxic protein found in the Alzheimer's brain during autopsy?

Dr. C. Kutscher, Psychopharmacology, relates more educational information in "Notes on Chapter 4 Carlson," he says, "Examples of ligands which have been especially well studied are dopamine, norepinephine, serotonin, epinephrine [adrenalin,] and acetylcholine. These are often called the "canonical transmitters. Neurochemists have found that many neurons contain a canonical transmitter along with an amino acid. The amino acids were found to be neurotransmitters also. Glutamate [or glutamic acid] is the prime excitatory neurotransmitter of the brain. It has four principle types of receptor sites, but the most widely studied is the NMDA receptor site" [Author- NMDA refers to, N-methyl-D-aspartate.]

Dr. Kutscher says, "The major inhibitory neurotransmitter is GABA. [Gama - aminobutyric acid.] It's binding to a receptor site is facilitated by drugs such as, alcohol, barbiturates and other drugs producing inhibition in the nervous system. Carlson's book suggests that these amino acids play the major role in neurotransmission and that the canonical transmitters are modulators. They modulate the rate of firing of neurons. So we see that drugs have strong effects on the brain, if they can change the way neurotransmitters bind to receptor sites in the nervous system and produce EPSPs and IPSPs."

What excellent explanatory information.

One thing that especially caught my eye here is the line that read, "Therefore we see that drugs" **[Author-I take this to mean possibly like combined chemical food and drink additives]** "have strong effects on the brain, if they can change the way neurotransmitters bind to receptor sites."

I want to track another thought that might be productive. *An article in the Houston Chronicle, Tuesday, Oct. 2, 2001, page 20a, written by Deborah Mann Lake, titled,* "Focus: Multiple Sclerosis, [MS] cool fashion." *Ms. Lake relates in the article that,* "A special vest reduces heat and symptoms for sufferers of MS. A gentleman in League City, Texas, wears a cooling vest lined with tubing, which circulates cool water to reduce MS symptoms."

Dr. Victor Rivera, Deputy Chief of Neurology, at the Methodist Hospital, stated in the article that, "We've known for years that an elevated temperature, whether environmental or from a fever, slows down the conduction of the nerve impulses in the areas affected by MS. If you can keep a person cool, it helps with symptoms."

An article published in the New York Times, titled, MS symptoms said to lessen with cooler temperatures says, "Researchers in the Netherlands and Russia found in their experimenting with cool vests and cap that, nitric oxide levels dropped when patients were cooled. Because nitric oxide is known to block conduction in nerve cells damaged by the disease, further research may lead to treatments that mimic the effects of cooling."

Ok! My understanding from these two articles is, when a person has MS and the temperature rises two things occur, nerve conduction slows in the effected areas and nitric oxide levels are elevated. Cooling reverses the situation.

It is my contention that amino acids and proteins may be altered and become toxic by inter-action with the combined effects of methyl-eugenol, ethyl-vanillin, and emulsifiers.

In talking elevated temperatures, I believe you will find the following to be very interesting.

The web site,

http://www.confex.com/ift/99annual/abstracts/3603.htm *relates information titled,* "Kinetics of interaction of vanillin with amino acids and peptides in model systems." *W. Chobpattana and Associates says,* "Vanillin, an aromatic aldehyde is a major compound of vanilla that is widely used as a food flavorant. Many studies have shown that interaction of vanillin and protein can cause flavor loss." *The team further relates that,* "Even though the vanillin-protein interactions have been extensively studied few studies on the kinetics of vanillin-amino acids or peptides have been reported."

Merriam-Webster's Collegiate Dictionary, describes the defination of kinetics as, "The change in a physical or chemical system."

Regarding MS, in the above article, concerning heat, I found the following information interesting. *W. Chobpattana, I. J. Leon and J. S. Smith, Department of Animal Sciences and Industry, Kansas State University, Manhattan, KS. State in their test results that,* "The reaction rate of vanillin-amino acids/peptides were accelerated as temperature increased. The rate constants were highest for pentalysine, followed by lysine, phenylalanine, glutathione, cysteine and aspartame."

Follow closely here, this is important. The reaction rate of vanillin, amino acids / peptides was accelerated as temperature increased. So, the point here is, vanillin coming into contact with protein, amino acids and peptides lose flavor. I see this as breaking down biochemically. When the temperature was increased, the breakdown was accelerated.

My logical mind asks this question:

Is vanillin a major culprit in other neurodegenerative diseases when the biochemical system ages, or because genetic mutations allows oxidation of minerals and trace elements?

The stronger ethyl vanillin in desserts is a triple strength oxidizer.

CHAPTER EIGHT:
ALCOHOL AND
B-VITAMINS

In this chapter, I want to write about the affects alcohol can have on my body. Alcohol can destroy B-vitamins, which I need for good mental health.

Consider how important the following B-Vitamin functions are.

Vitamin B-1 [Thiamine,] helps in the production of acetylcholine. Acetylcholine production is deficient in Alzheimer's disease. Vitamin B-1 is necessary to process glucose and is needed for the nervous system [as in neurodegeneration of the brain.]

According to The Real Vitamin and Mineral Book, "Vitamin B-1 plays an essential role in the metabolism of carbohydrates, a major source of energy in our cells." *The book goes on to say,* "This probably explains why the cells of the brain and the nervous system – are extremely sensitive to carbohydrate metabolism – are the first to show signs of thiamine deficiency."

Vitamin B-2, [Riboflavin] is involved in oxidation-reduction. [Anti-oxidants are prescribed to treat Alzheimer's.] Vitamin B-2 helps in the breakdown of carbohydrates. Breaking down carbohydrates is necessary for the production of adenosine triphosphate [ATP]. This chemical supplies the energy that powers our cells, [research indicates the Alzheimer brain is low on energy.] *According to the book titled, "Foods to Heal By," written by Barry Fox Ph.D,* "Good amounts of vitamin B-2 [5-10 milligrams per day] seem to encourage a better memory."

The Mosby Medical Encyclopedia, describes
Vitamin B-2 as, "A yellow crystal-like, heat-stable part of the B vitamin complex. It is not stored in any large amount in the body and must be gotten from the diet."

Vitamin B-3 [Niacin,] is involved in the breakdown of food. In order for food to be metabolized, it must be broken down. [How many Alzheimer's patients have you seen that passed away over weight?] When Mother passed away she was skin and bones.

Vitamin B-5 [Pantothenic acid,] "Releases energy from food necessary to make vitamin D hormones, and red blood cells *says the book titled, "The Complete Idiot's Guide to Vitamins and Minerals." Continuing on, co-author Dr. Alan H. Pressman says,* "You need pantothenic acid to make two crucial coenzymes: coenzyme A [CoA] and acyl carrier protein [ACP.]" *The book titled, "Total Nutrition from the Mount Sinai School of Medicine" says,* "Pantothenic acid is involved in the metabolism of lipids, carbohydrates and some amino acids."

Vitamin B-6 [Pyridoxine,] is needed for red blood cell production and helps to metabolize foods. Red blood cells are needed to carry oxygen to the brain. Oxygen is necessary to produce adenosine triphosphate [ATP]. "The main job of pyridoxine is shuffling around your amino acids to make the 5,000-plus proteins your body needs to run properly," *says Ms. Sheila Buff, Co-author of, "The Complete Idiot's Guide to Vitamins and Minerals."*

The Mosby Medical Encyclopedia, says, "A need for more pyridoxine occurs during aging."

Vitamin B-7 [Biotin,] "Releases energy from food" *says the book titled, "Vitamins and Minerals."*

The book titled, "Foods to Heal By," states that, "Biotin was actually the first vitamin to be discovered, in 1901. This was in the early days of vitamin research, however, before we really understood vitamins, so this strange new substance was given the name "Bios," meaning life."

Vitamin B-9 [Folic acid,] "Is needed for cell growth and reproduction," *says the Mosby Medical Encyclopedia. Continuing on the Encyclopedia says,* "It functions with vitamins B-12 and C in the breakdown of proteins and in the making of hemoglobin." Folic acid is also involved in the making of hydrochloric acid in the stomach.

Dr. Shari Lieberman and Nancy Bruning, relate in their book titled, "The Real Vitamin and Mineral Book" that, "Folic acid, also known as folate or folacin, was identified and named in the 1940's. In one of its most important roles folic acid works closely with vitamin B-12 in the metabolism of amino acids and the synthesis of proteins, and in the production of genetic material [RNA and DNA.]" *Continuing on, the book says,* "Thus, it is vital to healthy cell division and replication and to tissue growth. A number of its therapeutic uses are related to this function."

"Vitamin B-12 [Cobalamin,] is needed for DNA synthesis, and is important for proper nerve function. Vitamin B-12 is needed to make all blood cells and a deficiency eventually produces severe anemia" *says the book titled, "Total Nutrition." Reporting further, the book says,* "B-12 is necessary to make nerve sheaths and therefore, for proper nerve function." *Continuing on the book says,* "Since appreciable amounts of B-12 can be stored in the liver it may take years for a dietary deficiency to become apparent." Since B-12 deficiency is common in elderly people and Alzheimer's is a problem for older persons, I find that last line interesting, don't you?

So you can see, all the water soluble B-vitamins are extremely important, to not only, our mental health, but to our health in general. Alcohol in excess destroys B-vitamins. Enzymes need vitamins, because they act as co-factors in catalyzing rapid biochemical reactions.

Follow along with me here, I want to show you something. Consider that the essential amino acid tryptophan cannot be manufactured by the body, but, must be acquired from our food. Tryptophan is the precursor of the neurotransmitter serotonin and in the process niacin [vitamin B-3] is produced. When one understands that B-3 is necessary in food metabolism and important to the nervous system and serotonin is involved in depression and in the production of melatonin [necessary for the immune system and for sleep function]. When one comprehends this, then it does not take a rocket scientist to understand that at the headwaters of tryptophan there is a dam.

[A compromised tryptophan mutant.] <u>Think nitrogen inhibition.</u>

A deficiency of the combined vitamins B-6 [pyridoxine,] B-9 [folic acid,] and B-12 [cobalamin,] can result in increased homocysteine in the blood. A poison builds up reducing blood flow. Some Alzheimer's treatments are designed to increase the blood flow.

Think how destructive excess Alcohol is to Vitamins:

Alcohol can reduce the absorption of zinc, glucose, amino acids, vitamins and other important essentials. Alcohol can block the metabolism of vitamins. Alcohol use may block absorption of nutrients that my body and brain needs. The Immune system functions are impaired by alcohol related malnutrition. One would think that alcohol is totally taboo, especially where Alzheimer's disease is concerned. But think again. Consider the test results reported in the following newspaper article.

A study on the effects of alcohol and Alzheimer's disease shows, "Moderate drinking may block Alzheimer's disease" *says the Houston Chronicle newspaper USA. The Chronicle reports that,* "A study published in the, Lancet Medical Journal found that daily moderate consumption of alcohol might ward off Alzheimer's disease and other types of dementia." *The article states,* "Experts say, between one and three drinks a day is the key. Scientists at Erasmus University, in Rotterdam, the Netherlands conducted a six-year study of 5,395 people aged 55 and over who did not have signs of dementia." *The article relates that,* "By the end of the study in 1999, 197 of the participants developed Alzheimer's or another form of dementia." *Meir Stampfer professor of nutrition and epidemiology, Harvard School of Public Health, who was quoted in the article said,* "For people who drink moderately, this is another indication that they are not doing any harm."

Boy Howdy! That's like telling this "Ole Texas Boy" that up is down. "Well! Buddy have a drink." After reading the article, I walked around for a couple days thinking, those people are nuts if they believe that.

After I settled down, I started to think in depth about it. The first thing I looked at was the percentage of folks that got Alzheimer's or dementia. According to my calculations, about 8% of us are at risk. 8 % of those tested would have come out to about 432 people, but only 197 were affected with Alzheimer's or dementia.

I tried to reason this out. I know I am right, so what is going on here? Somehow, these numbers had to fit in with my hypothesis of what I know is causing Alzheimer's disease. I know from my research and testing on myself, that my Alzheimer's dementia is being caused when my body no longer can process eugenol, methyl-eugenol, vanillin, ethyl vanillin or propylene glycol-ethyl vanillin. [Artificial flavors, emulsifiers and a solvent.]

I think I have found the answer.

On *Rhodia's web site,*
http://www.food.us.rhodia.com/brochures/romexpvn/page4.asp, it is stated, "Ethyl vanillin is soluble in alcohol." When a substance is diluted, then its effect is diminished, and tests results should show fewer people affected, which the tests confirmed.

Something to ponder here, alcohol in our blood reaches the brain and we become "tipsy." Since these compounds will mix with alcohol, can they also enter our brain?

As long as were talking methyl-eugenol and ethyl-vanillin [artificial flavors,] I have some questions regarding what happens in my body when an emulsifier is added to this mix. Adding an emulsifier to methyl-eugenol and or ethyl-vanillin increased dementia, confusion, and Alzheimer's symptoms, in testing on myself many times over.

Although methyl-eugenol and ethyl-vanillin will dissolve in alcohol, they are only slightly soluble in water. When I think about emulsifiers and how they allow oils and water to mix as in margarine or ice cream, the question is this, do emulsifiers allow methyl-eugenol, ethyl-vanillin to mix with water in our bodies when they wouldn't normally, and, if they can mix with water, what bad things are they doing to amino acids, proteins, enzymes, cells, hormones, neurotransmitters and the processing of nutrients?

Can these chemical additives, mix with water, enter the cell effecting mitochondria, the cells energy supplier of ATP?

How about the cells nucleus and DNA. Can these combined chemical additives be the source of gene mutation that block or alters the proper formulation of protein? Is this one of the culprits of over production in amyloid beta 1-42 peptide that contributes to toxic plaque in Alzheimer's brain cells? Both amyloid beta 40 and amyloid beta 42 are cleaved from amyloid precursor protein [APP.] Amyloid beta 42 is the most toxic form.

In my opinion, based on several years of Alzheimer's testing on myself, the problem with Alzheimer's disease involves two combined chemical additives [artificial flavors combined with emulsifiers] in our food and drink, when they are placed in an elderly person's body.

CHAPTER NINE:
EUGENOL AND
ALCOHOL

Thinking of the multiple neurological degenerative diseases of the brain, common logic kick's in and I think, with all the highly educated neurological researchers working hard to find cures for these disease's, why are the researchers coming up short? These people are extremely bright. The only logical answer is, chemical compounds and the resulting kinetic interaction with amino acids and peptides have a way of masking their identify, or, scientists would have discovered the cause and cure of Alzheimer's disease long ago.

Phenol is one such chemical to consider.

Merriam-Webster's Collegiate Dictionary describes Phenol as, "A corrosive poisonous crystalline acidic compound C_6H_5OH present in coal tar and wood tar that in dilute solution is used as a disinfectant."

Vanillin is one chemical compound food additive distilled from eugenol, we should consider that contains phenol.

Vanillin:

April 2, 2002

According to an extra pure vanillin brochure from the web site, http:// www.food.us.rhodia.com/brochures/epv/page17.asp, "Vanillin is an interesting compound, possessing both a phenolic and aldehydic group and is capable of undergoing a number of different types of chemical reactions." *The site further states,* "Additional reactions are possible, due to the reactivity of the aromatic nucleus and exposure to air causes vanillin to oxidize slowly to vanillic acid." *The web site relates that,* "When vanillin is exposed to light in an alcoholic solution, a slow dimerisation takes place with the formation of dehydrodivanillin. This compound is also formed in other solvents." *The web site also states that,* "All three functional groups in vanillin are highly reactive," [Phenolic, aldehydic, and hydroxyl.

The Mosby Medical Encyclopedia Revised Edition, states that, "Air is composed of 78 % nitrogen, 21 % oxygen, almost 1 % argon and small amounts of carbon dioxide."

Here are my thoughts. Exposure to *air* causes vanillin to oxidize slowly to vanillic acid. Nitrogen binds with protein. Nitrogen and oxygen, *air* are carried in the bloodstream. The reason I mention this is I am recalling something I read. Let's go back to Gene, [chapter five] my childhood friend and his autopsy report. Something that caught my eye and may not mean anything, but, if we are to be successful with this endeavor we need to consider all possibilities. "Some chemical compounds are excreted in the urine."

Gene's autopsy report, states, "There is ulceration of the urethral meatus." Something in Gene's urine may have been destroying tissue. Could this have been vanillic acid, his aged immune system would not breakdown? I have several articles that speak of vanillic acid being flushed out of the body in urine, after the ingestion of foods containing vanillin.

Eugenol and vanillin are practically non-water-soluble. So, how do they get in urine? I believe the answer is emulsifiers. They allow water and oils to mix. Do we now enter a whole new world of possible health problems by allowing water-soluble and fat-soluble vitamins to go where they were not intended to go in an aged person's body?

According to Rhodia's web site, "Exposure to air causes vanillin to oxidize slowly to vanillic acid. When vanillin is exposed to light in an alcoholic solution, a slow dimerisation takes place with the formation of dehydrodivanillin. This compound is also found in other solvents." [Solvents like to dissolve.]

So to get dehydrodivanillin, we need vanillin, alcohol and light. Let's say, as an elderly person with an age-weakened immune and biochemical defense system, I eat a large bowl of vanilla ice cream made with artificial flavor [vanillin.] Now I have the vanillin. An emulsifier is also used in the making of ice cream. They also put vanilla extract in vanilla ice cream. Vanilla extract is made by, soaking vanilla beans in hot alcohol. I now have the vanillin and alcohol, plus the emulsifier.

All I need is the light, electromagnetic radiation [like the light that comes through our eyes] to produce "dehydrodivanillin" [solvent.]

When brain cells fire, this produces the energy needed to convert the vanillin to dehydrodivanillin, [solvent.] Think amyloid plaque.

Everyone is looking for the cause of the beta amyloid plaque. Isn't the above information the source of the plaque?

If these toxic chemicals overpower my age-weakened biochemical system, can this be the source of the toxic protein that forms beta amyloid plaque and tau tangles?

In my quest for answers, my reading and research has been enormous, to say the least. I have read of only a few studies involving vanillin. There are not many. In a few studies vanillic acid was found in the urine after ingesting vanillin.

However, I have never once read of dehydrodivanillin being excreted from the body. Could it be that it remains in the body if the immune system and biochemical defense system is weak, and cannot break it down? Another thought comes to mind here.

Could this also be the source of Amyloidosis?

Stedman's Medical Dictionary, describes Amyloidosis as, "A disorder marked by the deposition of amyloid in various organs and tissues of the body that may be associated with a chronic disease such as rheumatoid arthritis, tuberculosis or multiple myeloma."

Normally we think of light as entering the eye and we can see but there may be much more going on here. *According to the Mosby Medical Encyclopedia, Revised Edition,* "Light is radiant energy of the wavelength and frequency that stimulate visual receptor cells in the retina of the eye to produce nerve impulses that are perceived in the brain as vision."

After light enters the eye, it is collected by rods and cones on the retina. This electromagnetic radiation then travels by way of the optic nerve to an area near the center of the brain, where the pineal gland is located.

Amyloid plaque has now been found in the cataracts of Alzheimer's patients. Think light.

The Encyclopedia of Nutritional Supplements states that, "The pineal gland, a small pea sized gland at the base of the brain, has been a source of curiosity since antiquity. The ancient Greeks considered the pineal gland, the seat of the soul, a concept that was extended by the philosopher Descartes." Scientific research states that the pineal gland secretes melatonin. So as we age, develop Alzheimer's and have a problem sleeping, can this be caused by the bodies inability to use and convert the electromagnetic radiation [light] properly? Does this inhibit the pineal gland from producing the melatonin and thereby interfering with circadian rhythm [the body's internal clock?] The immune system utilizes melatonin, so if the body loses its ability to produce it, through electromagnetic radiation conversion, could this help to explain why the biochemical system ages in us older folks?

Was Gene's, "aged immune system" torpedoed by the toxic oxidizers, methyl-eugenol, ethyl-vanillin [artificial flavors] combined with emulsifiers, that his body could no longer process, resulting in his cognitive impairment, malnutrition and eventually his death?

Many works are being performed by our Creators light with its oscillating wavelength and vibrating frequencies, near the center of the brain.

CHAPTER TEN:
EXPOSED

What is causing this horrible Alzheimer's disease?

It has destroyed so many families worldwide, both emotionally and financially. In my opinion, Alzheimer's disease shows up when an age weakened immune system and biochemical defense system no longer can process two combined chemical compound additives found in our food and drink.

I classify eugenol, isoeugenol, methyl-eugenol,

Ethyl-vanillin and vanillin as one compound. I know they have different chemical formulas, but in testing on myself, I have concluded their effect on my brain cells is the same. We need to start at the source of one of the food and drink combined chemical additives [eugenol], which I believe is one cause of this problem.

Clove oil:

The following web site, http://193.51.164.11/htdocs/monographs/vol36/eugenol.html, says, "Eugenol, occurs widely as a component of essential oils and is a major constituent of clove oil. Used since the 19th Century as a flavoring agent in foods, pharmaceutical products and in dental materials."

7th Edition of McGraw-Hill Encyclopedias of Science and Technology, page 39 defines clove as, "The unopened flower bud of a small, conical, symmetrical evergreen tree, Eugenia Caryophyllata...of the Myrtle family." *The book goes on to say,* "The cloves are picked by hand and sun dried. Cloves, one of the most important and useful spices are strongly aromatic and have a pungent flavor. Cloves are used as a culinary spice for flavoring pickles, ketchup and sauces. Cloves are also used in medicine. 90 % of the clove production comes from Tanzania."

In my opinion, this eugenol problem is enormous for people with an age related weakened immune and biochemical defense system. I want to question it and other similar chemicals I believe caused my Alzheimer's disease. Eugenol is an oxidizer. Think antioxidants.

One web site that defines eugenol is,

http://www.scorecard.org/chemical-.../consumer-products.tcl?   edf_substance_id=97%2d53%2d it says, "Eugenol known by the Iupac [International Union of Pure and Applied Chemistry] name, 4 methoxy-4-allylphenol. Eugenol, is a clear colorless or sometimes, pale yellow liquid. It has a catalog Id number 000101 and a CAS number of 97-53-0."

The Great American Heritage Dictionary, Third Edition, 1996, describes eugenol as, "A colorless aromatic liquid C10 H12 O2, made from clove oil and used as a dental analgesic and in perfumery." Eugenol is an aromatic compound in artificial flavors. It is used in food and drinks because artificial flavors are cheap to produce compared to natural flavoring.

The web site, Webmd/Lycos-article-eugenol oil overdose regarding eugenol says, "Eugenol oil overdoses; poisonous ingredient actions, call poison control center from yellow pages."

July 25, 2000

More information is provided on **eugenol** from

The web site, http://www.ehs.cornell.edu/lrs/labels/Eugenol.html, as follows:

"Caution! Combustible!

CAS # 97-53-0

STATEMENT OF HAZARDS:

Skin and eye irritation. Liver damage. Local analgesia. Gastroenteritis. Peripheral vascular collapse.

PRECAUTIONARY STATEMENTS:

Avoid contact with skin and eyes. Do not breathe vapor.

FIRST AID:

Inhalation: If inhaled, remove to fresh air. If not breathing give artificial respiration. Skin: In case of contact, immediately wash skin with soap and water. Eye: In case of contact, immediately flush with plenty of water for at least 15 minutes."

Eugenol and its derivatives can be found in our food, drink and in some medications used as artificial flavors.

There are very few studies on Eugenol and Humans:

The web site,

http://193.51164.11/htdocs/monographs/vol36/eugenol.html, relates this information regarding, "Eugenol; 5.3 human data.

No case report or epidemiological study of the carcinogenicity of eugenol to humans was available to the working group." The web site says,

EVALUATION:

In the absence of epidemiological data, no evaluation could be made of the carcinogenicity of eugenol to humans."

According to The Environmental Defense Scorecard, "If the basic tests to check on the toxicity of a chemical have not been conducted, or if the results are not publicly, available, current laws tend to treat that chemical as if it were perfectly safe."

Regarding neurotoxicity references; *the following web site, http://www.scorecard.org/health-effects/references.tcl? Short_hazard_ name=neuro 10/21/01. States,* "There is no generally accepted source for an authoritative list of chemicals that are recognized to cause neurotoxicity."

One thing confusing the identities of eugenol and its counterpart vanillin, [I use the word counterpart, because, vanillin being distilled from eugenol is actually an extension of eugenol,] is that, there are multiple names for eugenol, vanillin and other chemical compounds. Eugenol, is an electron acceptor, the following represent only some of the synonyms for eugenol.

4-alkylphenol.

4 hydroxybenzyl alcohol phenol.

2-methoxy-4- 2-propenyl.

Regarding eugenol, the following web site

http://www.hclrss.demon.co.uk/methyl_eugenol. States that, "The name methyl eugenol is approved by the Entomological Society of America. Notes: There is no ISO [International Standards Organization] common name for this substance."

**Multiple names for eugenol are confusing the issue.
"I will show this by listing some of them."**
The NTP Chemical Repository [Radian Corporation,]
Lists eugenol synonyms as,
"Eugenol synonyms:
4-Allylcatechol-2-methyl ether
4-Allylguaiacol
4-Allyl-1-hydroxy-2-methoxybenzene
4-Allyl-2-methoxyphenol
Caryophyllic acid
Eugenic acid:
1-Hydroxy-2-methoxy-4-prop-2-enylbenzene
2-Methoxy-4-prop-2-enylphenol
2-Methoxy-4- (2-propenyl) phenol
P-Eugenol
1, 3, 4-Eugenol
1-Hydroxy-2-methoxy-4-allylbenzene
P-Allylguaiacol
Fa 100
Fema no. 2467
4-hydroxy-3-methoxyallylbenzene
2-Methoxy-1-hydroxy-4-allylbenzene
Nci-c50453
Synthetic eugenol
Phenol, 4-allyl-2-methoxy
Phenol, 2-methoxy-4- (2-propenyl)-
1-allyl-4-hydroxy-3-methoxybenzene
Allylguaiacol
1-Hydroxy-4-allyl-2-methoxybenzene
1-Hydroxy-2-methoxy-4-propenylbenzene
2-Methoxy-4- (2-propen-1-yl) phenol.

I could have said, "There are 25 other synonyms for eugenol." The point is, This "Dangerous Duo," eugenol and vanillin, have multiple identities and they may be a serious problem for the 8 % of us older folks at risk for mild cognitive impairment [MCI] that may lead to Alzheimer's dementia.

Are you confused? Will the "Real Eugenol" please stand up? Eugenol is sold all over the world. Alzheimer's disease is also all over the world. Duh!

Japanese sales of eugenol:

The web site,
"http://www.chemical-metal.co.jp/jcs/product/e/e100.html lists eugenol
as, P-hydroxy-m-methoxy-2-propenyl benzene
Eugenic acid 2-methoxy-4- [2-propenyl] phenol
4-allylguacol
Japan chemical search."

Chinese sales of vanillin:

The web site
http://www.tradezone.com/tradesites/girasole.html states that, "We are a manufacture from China. We produce and export food additive vanillin, other vanillin, ethyl vanillin, etc.
Zhonhua Chemical Industry Co., ltd."

Think all these different names for eugenol is confusing. As Jimmy Durante said,

" Youse ain't seen nothin yet."

Pay attention to the following:

The Enviromental Defense Scorecard web site
http://www.scorecard.org/chemicalprofiles/summary.tcl
? edf_substance_id=97-53-0
Relates the following information,
"Eugenol; chemical health hazard.
Suspected gastrointestinal or liver toxicant, neurotoxicant."

"Neurotoxicant?"

Like toxic to neurons, like neurons in the brain, like maybe Alzheimer's toxic amyloid plaque that kills brain cells. Is oxidation leaching out the iron and aluminum from containers? When brain cells fire, do they dissolve toxic protein into amyloid plaque that destroys brain cells? What is that I am hearing in the distance ...mutated enzymes...altered proteins?

The following web site,
http://ntpdb.niehs.nih.gov/ntp_reports/ntp_chem_h&s/ntp_chem9/
radian97-53-0.tx relates that, "Eugenol; is used in the production of
iso-eugenol for the manufacture of vanillin."

There are other uses for vanillin in our food supply.

The web site, http://www.theeyeofnewt.com/store/html/items/specialty
product says, "Vanilla powder is defined as, a specialty product used as a
flavoring agent in candy, beverages, foods and animal feed. Used as an
aroma additive in cosmetics."

Vanillin also has many different chemical names:

The following information regarding vanillin, is published on the,
UCSD, Chemistry & Biochemistry web site,
http://chem-courses.ucsd.edu/coursepages/uglabs/msds/vanillin-info.
html, and says,

"Vanillin synonyms:
M-anisaldehyde.
4-hydroxy- benzaldehyde.
4-hydroxy-3-methoxy.
P-hydroxy-m-methoxybenzaldehyde.
4-hydroxy-3-methoxybenzaldhyde.
Lioxin.
3-methoxy-4-hydroxybenzaldehyde.
Protocatechualdehyde.
Methyl vanilla.
Vanillaldehyde.
Vanillic aldehyde.
P- Vanillin.
Vanilline.
Zimco."

I want to repeat this. "Vanillin exposed to air converts to vanillic
acid. We have air, which is oxygen and nitrogen in our bodies."

The following web site, http://www.alfa.com/cgi-bin/odc_webcat/jump.
cgi? File=msds/a12074.html

Says, "Vanillic acid; molecular formula: $C_8 H_8 O_4$

Alternative names: 4-hydroxy-3-methoxybenzoic acid
Material Safety Data Sheet a12074."

Handling and storage of vanillic acid:
"Respiratory;
Avoid inhalation of product.
Eye;
Avoid eye contact.
Protect from moisture
Hands and Body;
Irritant product.
Avoid skin contact.
Storage;
Protect from moisture"

Protect from moisture?
The Funk & Wagnalls-Atlas of the Body, states that, "Water is about
60% of the male or female's body weight, on average."
***Therefore, if we ingest vanillin how do we protect it from
moisture?***
Boy – Howdy!
As William Bendix, "Life of Riley" said,
"What a revolting development this is."
Vanillin:
60% of vanillin is used in food and beverages.
20 % is used for flavor and fragrances. 5-10% of vanillin is used for
intermediates for pharmaceuticals.
More multiple chemical names for vanillin:
The web site,
*http://lanminds.com/wilworks/bbchem/1500chmv.html   lists   more
names for vanillin as,*

Chemical	CAS Number
Vanilla tincture	8047-24-3
Vanillic acid	121-34-6

Vanillin	121-33-5
Vanillin acetate	881-68-5
Vanillin isobutyrate	20665-85-4
Vanillin propylene glycol--acetal	68527-74-2

**Are you confused? Will the "Real Vanillin" please
stand up? Vanillin is sold all over the world.
Alzheimer's disease is also all over the world.
Another duh!**

Rhodia, one major International company that manufactures vanillin, published the following information on their web site. "For the years 1993-95, the estimated worldwide production of vanillin was 10,000 tones per year."

Over the years, Rhodia has expanded production on the International scene. "In 1970, Rhodia opened a plant at St-Fons South Lyon, France. A second plant, a few years later was opened at New Brunswick, New Jersey, USA. In 1978, another vanillin plant was opened at St-Fons North Lyon France."

"In 1981, the St-Fons North plant in France began production of Rhodiarome, extra pure ethyl vanillin, 2.6 times the strength of vanillin."

"In 1990, they opened a plant to produce, extra pure ethyl vanillin and ethyl vanillin, at Baton Rouge, Louisiana, USA."

Rhodia states, "Rhodiarome [ethyl vanillin] is used in cakes, pastries, biscuits, chocolates, confections and sweets." *They also state that,* "This product is a substitute for vanillin. It is considered to have 3 to 4 times the flavoring strength of vanillin."

I do not believe that vanillin is a problem for younger people. My work shows, it only becomes a problem, when the biochemical system in our body weakens from aging.

In chapter 12, titled *"Melatonin," we will find reference to the work by Dr. Jose Luchsinger, lead author of the study at Columbia University. He* said, "People, who consumed the most calories and fats, faced double the risk of developing Alzheimer's."

For those who think calories and fats cause Alzheimer's, ask yourself this question. Why don't kids develop Alzheimer's dementia? They gorge themselves with pastries, candy and ice creams! In my opinion,

"It's because their biochemical system is young, healthy and strong and it will process out these combined chemical additives in their food and drinks, without any problems."

However, in my opinion, it's not the calories and fats that cause Alzheimer's, they just happen to be in the same foods that eugenol, methyl-eugenol, ethyl-vanillin and emulsifiers are, especially propylene-glycol, ethyl-vanillin.

Packaging;

On Rhodia's web site, http://www.food.us.rhodia.com/datasheets/template1.asp? PID=222 they advise, "Containers should be closed and kept away from light, heat and moisture. It is recommended to avoid using iron or steel containers."

Avoid using iron or steel containers?

Vanillin, placed in these iron or steel containers and exposed to light [like the kind that comes through our eyes] can leach out some of the iron or steel from the containers by the process of oxidation. Think oxidative stress and mis-folded proteins that cause neurodegenerative diseases.

Regarding Vanillin:

The web site, http://www.foodproductdesign.com/archive/1998/0898cs.html reports that, "Vanillin can react with iron to form a pinkish-colored compound." Iron residue has been found in Alzheimer's patient's brains after death.

Regarding excess iron, *the alzforum web site, http://www.alzforum.org/members/resourses/journal abstract.html states that,* "Iron accumulation in the brain is a consistent observation in Alzheimer's disease." **Think eugenol-vanillin oxidized iron.**

Vanillin is also found in coal tar and crude petroleum. It can be distilled out of the tar, usually guaiacol. It is called ethyl-vanillin. Ethyl-vanillin is three times as strong as regular vanillin.

The following web site, http://www.inchem.org/documents/sids/sids/sids5b06.htm states regarding vanillin, "The acute toxicity to fish has been tested in fathead minnow. It was observed that the fish stopped schooling, became hypoactive, swam at the surface and lost equilibrium prior to death." *The site says,* "There are no data available on the chronic toxicity to fish."

Older people eat a lot of ice cream. Most of it contains vanillin or artificial flavor, distilled from eugenol the aromatic compound. [Methyl-eugenol and ethyl-vanillin.] Eating ice cream is not the only way those of us who are at risk for Alzheimer's may be getting cognitive impairment and dementia. Most all candy bars have these ingredients, as do most soft drinks and nearly all bakery products.

Regarding products containing ethyl-vanillin: the web site*, Ethyl procatechuric aldehyde. 3-ethoxy-4-hydroxybenzaldehyde http://www. chemical-metal.co.jp/jcs/product/e/e038.html,*

Relates three items that contain ethyl-vanillin:
Ethovan.
Bourbonal.
Vanirom.

Think how confusing all these chemical compounds and their kinetic interactions with amino acids, and peptides look to a bright neuroresearcher trying to solve Alzheimer's. These compounds have been obstacles for Alzheimer's researchers for 100 years. That is how long it has been, since Dr. Alzheimer diagnosed the first case of Alzheimer's disease.

A young healthy biochemical system will deliver a knock out punch to these combined chemical food and drink additives. That is why there may be no memory problems with these combined chemical additives until we get old. Then our immune and biochemical defense system becomes weakened and our memory may be affected by "Trace Mineral Deficiency," creating a need to re-supply certain atomic elements.

For more information on this, visit our web site at
www.zapalzheimers.com.

I have eaten these combined chemical additives in food and drink all my life, and remained very, very, healthy and mentally sharp. When I reached 65 years of age, these combined chemical additives started to cause memory problems for me. The same kind of problems that killed my mother. This horrible disease called "Alzheimer's dementia."

Rhodia, further states on their web site, http://www.food.us.rhodia. com/brochures/romexpvn/page2.asp that, "Extra pure ethyl vanillin is 2.6

times stronger in flavor than vanillin." *They say,* "3.3 times stronger in milk solutions."

Critics say, "Hey! We put 100 people in a room, fed them vanillin. It only affected eight people, this is inconclusive." I say, "Quite the contrary. Since only 8 % of us older folks may be affected by Alzheimer's; [because of an age weakening biochemical and immune system] 100% of the people at risk for Alzheimer's may have been affected. Those may be the people whose body no longer would process the combined chemical food and drink additives."

Vanilla extract is added to vanillin to increase the flavor and make it taste more like real vanilla. This adds more vanillin and sometimes as much as 35% alcohol. See chapter 8 titled, "Alcohol and B-Vitamins."

Being unaware of the multiple types of eugenol and vanillin, in the beginning of my testing made it hard to isolate the cause of my cognitive impairment, but, I kept after it. Failure was never an option. I never recall thinking I could not figure this out.

The plan was to get from point A to point B. The requirements were to spend whatever amount of time it took. Eventually, it became over seven years of reading medical books, praying and researching the web practically day and night, seven days a week.

This does not include the six years I struggled to understand what the six numbers meant. I knew, if I didn't want to die like my poor Mother, slobbering over the side of a wheel chair, unable to function mentally, I had one chance. I had to figure out the cause of this Alzheimer's disease. What I did not understand at the time, was the *"six numbers"* that occurred years earlier was on a collision course with my process of elimination diet to isolate the cause of my memory problems.

The odds of choosing the correct six numbers *["six elements"]* that are involved in Alzheimer's dementia are over 2.5 billion to one. [See the odds calculator in chapter 5.]

Scientific research supports the six atomic elements. This information can be found in chapter 17, titled, *"Conclusion, Putting It All Together."*

If I raise the ire of companies that manufacture alcohol, artificial flavors, eugenol, vanillin and emulsifiers, I want to clarify my position here. I am not saying, do not eat artificially flavored food and drink containing these substances.

I am saying, my age-weakened biochemical system no longer can process these combined chemical additives that are in certain food and drink. They were causing me a problem. The problem was severe Alzheimer's symptoms like Mother had.

I have become at risk for Alzheimer's because, certain elements in my body are being oxidized and disarmed, by the combined effects of chemical additives in my food and drink. <u>*Replacing the "six elements" on a continual basis solves my problem and blocks the effects of the combined chemical additives.*</u>

Agents of the immune system named Microglia, protect the brain. I believe certain elements are being inhibited and microglia can not function. Maybe the sticky toxic protein being dissolved by these combined chemicals traps microglia, stopping their function.

Someone has been watching this suffering and searching for answers to Alzheimer's disease for almost a century now. My guess is, in the final analysis, he figured we needed some help.

You should discuss these things with your doctor. He or she should be consulted on your health problems. They are the ones in charge here; I'm just telling you what worked on this 72 year old man. I mean I was able to write this book, Right!

Have you ever stopped to think about this? In the later stages of Alzheimer's disease, the patient loses the ability to pray to our Creator. <u>How can one ask for guidance and forgiveness if one cannot think progressively and recall from memory that we have a Creator?</u>

CHAPTER ELEVEN:
EUGENOL - VANILLIN
AND EMULSIFIERS

Based on years of research and three years of testing on myself, my findings are that Alzheimer's disease, and probably other forms of dementia, present themselves when the body will no longer process the combined chemical compounds methyl-eugenol, and ethyl-vanillin [artificial flavors] when combined with emulsifiers.

Does it concern you that they are putting eugenol in our foods?

May 23, 2000, the following web site, http://darkwing.uoregon. edu/~sshapiro/pemphigus/phenolics.html,_states, "Eugenol, is the main constituent of natural oils like carnation, clove, and cinnamon. It is used extensively in food flavorings. This compound is used in yeast production, in the manufacture of vanillin, in dental practice, and in perfumery." *Continuing on, the web site says,* "Eugenol is highly toxic in concentrated form. There is a strong suspicion that it is a major contributor to chronic urticaria [Hives] and is a strong nerve stimulator." *The site further says,* "Eugenol is an example of an aromatic compound found in a variety of foodstuffs." *The web site also states,* "An individual may be exposed to this aromatic by eating cloves, by inhaling certain perfumes, by eating candy to which it has been added or by chewing certain gums."

Scientists are studying the toxic amyloid plaque that is destroying brain cells in patients who have Alzheimer's disease. In my opinion, eugenol, vanillin and ethyl-vanillin play a major role in the formation of amyloid plaque, based on my testing.

Eugenol is highly toxic in concentrated form.

Think about this. They do a few tests measuring the effects of eugenol on our bodies and they say, "ok! Just a little eugenol is not toxic to humans as long as it is not in concentrated form." Let me ask you this question, if the aged biochemical system in our bodies loses the ability to process this eugenol chemical out of our bodies <u>could it not accumulate to the concentrated form where it would then be toxic?</u>

The following information details where Methyl-eugenol is added: "Federal Register: March five, 2001, volume. 66, no. 43. Notices. Pages 13334 - 13338.
Department of Health and Human Services.

Public Health Service
Methyl-eugenol

Reg. No. 93 - 15 - 2

Formula: C11H14O2." *It is further stated that,* "Methyl- eugenol, are flavoring agents used in jellies, baked goods, nonalcoholic beverages, chewing gum, candy and ice cream. Also used as fragrance for many perfumes, lotions, detergents and soaps." *It says,* "Motion to list methyl-eugenol as reasonably anticipated to be a human carcinogen passed by a vote of 9 yes to 1 no. The National Toxicology Program [NTP]"

There is one problem here!

The Department of Health and Human Services has listed, "Methyl-eugenol as reasonably anticipated to be a human carcinogen." Others claim it is a neurotoxicant. But the listed ingredients on wrappers of cakes, pastries, candy bars and ice cream labels are not methyl-eugenol, but vanillin and or artificial flavors. The public may hear caution about methyl-eugenol, but does not know caution about vanillin, when in reality, methyl-eugenol and ethyl-vanillin are almost identical chemical compounds. Some foods also contain emulsifiers.

When I tested on myself, searching to isolate the chemical that really put "The Gidyap" in my accelerated Alzheimer's symptoms. I discovered that ingesting foods with double emulsifiers combined with ethyl-vanillin, [double and triple strength vanillin] increased my cognitive impairment and dementia, big time.

The Emulsifier:

The on-line Medical Dictionary, describes the Emulsifier as, "A substance, which can be used to produce an emulsion out of two liquids that normally, cannot be mixed together, [such as oil and water.] Emulsifiers are common in foods to maintain consistency within puddings, powders, etc."

One of the emulsifiers I am most concerned with is propylene glycol. Combined with triple strength vanillin, it becomes propylene-glycol, ethyl-vanillin. This product is used in a great many desserts. My findings are when I ingest this product, it overpowers my age weakened biochemical defense system. This triggers memory loss, confusion, and loss of ability to think progressively. <u>Before,</u> I reached 65 years of age; propylene-glycol and ethyl-vanillin caused me no ill affects what so ever, as far as I know.

Stedman's Medical Dictionary, describes Propylene as, "A flammable gas derived from processing petroleum hydrocarbon and used in organic synthesis, also called propene."

Listing glycol separately, Stedman's Medical Dictionary, describes Glycol *as,* "Any of various alcohols containing two hydroxyl groups."

Mosby's Medical Nursing and Allied Health Dictionary, describes *Propylene-glycol as,* "A colorless viscous liquid used as a solvent in the preparation of certain medications," *Further describing propylene-glycol Mosby's says,* "It also inhibits the growth of fungi and microorganisms and is used commercially as an anti-freeze."

Merriam-Webster's Dictionary describes Propylene-glycol as, "A sweet hygroscopic viscous liquid C3H8O2 made especially from propylene and used especially as an anti-freeze and solvent, and in brake fluids."

In my opinion, 92 % of the population is not having memory problems from propylene-glycol and ethyl-vanillin.

What about the other 8% of us elderly?

So, one might say, dementia may be reflected in the elderly by their eating habits. Read the study in chapter 12 titled, "Melatonin," on calories, fats and Alzheimer's.

For example, I am at risk for Alzheimer's because, I love sweets. When I go to the bakery, I get the whole ball of wax that will increase my dementia, by eating their products. Donuts, rolls, and other baked goods. Most of these are made using, propylene-glycol and ethyl-vanillin. [Methyl-eugenol, ethyl-vanillin and an emulsifier.] Also included in almost all these bakery products is vanilla extract. Now, more alcohol and vanillin are present.

I want to clarify something here. In my opinion, if I was younger and my immune and biochemical defense system was still strong, these chemicals would not cause me any Alzheimer's symptoms, as I believe, they do not cause any memory problems for 92 % of the public.

I believe when we age, the immune system and the biochemical defense system weaken. When my body can no longer process these combined chemicals, then Alzheimer's dementia presents itself. My findings are methyl-eugenol, ethyl-vanillin, [artificial flavors] combined with emulsifiers, may be a serious problem for us older folks.

I am at risk of Alzheimer's because, my age related immune and biochemical defense system, has weakened, and will no longer process these chemical additives in my food and drink. I believe they were responsible for Mother's Alzheimer's disease. I knew her diet. She loved sweets and desserts that contained these chemicals. Mother almost never drank alcohol, but, she used a lot of vanilla extract in her baking which contained the alcohol and more vanillin.

These combined chemicals are inhibiting the "six elements," my brain needs to function correctly. Let me repeat this. It gets interesting. When I replace the "six elements," on a regular basis, I can eat the bakery products, candy, ice cream, soft drinks and other things that contain these chemical additives, like I used to, and my mind stays clear as ever. The odds of choosing the correct "six elements," from over 114 elements, in "The Periodic Table of Elements" that may reverse Alzheimer's disease, is over two billion to one.

The web site, <u>*http://www.inchem.org/documents/jecfa/jecmono/v35j*</u> <u>*07.htm*</u> says, "Ethyl vanillic acid; [3-ethoxy-4-hydroxybenzoic acid] not a normal constituent of human urine, has been identified in the urine of humans known to have ingested vanilla-flavored foodstuffs."

In another area, "big money has worked its magic." European legislation no longer requires artificial flavoring to be mentioned on the product packaging.

Presto - "Hoccus-Poccus" - It disappeared!

The word "flavoring" is now sufficient.

"Aye matie" did ye know lad?

We's got "vanillin sugar," and aye laddie, we's got

"Vanillin butter" also.

If'n yore in Thu land o Thu "Queen Mum," Tis "sneeky vanillin" now.

Vanillin, used as a starting material:

I was surprised to learn, drugs produced to treat some diseases, use a starting material of guess what? Vanillin. Is this a problem for an older person with an age weakened immune system? Certainly, the pharmaceutical companies are not aware of this. Someone should tell them.

Vanillin is incompatible with Iron and Zinc:

From the web site, http://webbook.nist.gov/cgi/cbook.cgi? Id=c148538&units=si "Is information regarding O-Vanillin, [2-hydroxy-3-methoxybenzaldehyde.] *The National Institute of Standards and Technology, [NIST] states,* "This chemical is incompatible with iron, zinc, ferric chloride, and potassium permanganate." Located on page two dated, November 22, 2000.

Incompatible with Iron and Zinc?

The Mosby Medical Encyclopedia defines Iron [Fe,] "As a common metallic element needed to make hemoglobin. Oxygen and iron carrying compound in the blood." *The Encyclopedia further describes Zinc [Zn] as,* "An essential nutrient in the body."

From the above information, we see that vanillin is not compatible with iron and zinc. Zinc is a major player in the sodium potassium pump. This is how ions are pumped in and out of the nerve cell. We also see how important iron and zinc are to the biochemical function of our bodies. Iron supplies the oxygen to the brain and the zinc is essential for nutrition.

I don't know about you, but when I read this, I have to wonder,

What in the Sam Hill is going on here?

If the iron [number 26] is inhibited, then doesn't it need to be replaced in order to correct the deficiency? The iron is being oxidized along with other oxidized metals, and winds up in the beta amyloid plaque found in the Alzheimer's brain.

I believe neuroresearcher Dr. Ashley Bush et, al; are on the right track with their patented clioquinol which involves metal chelating [the removal of metals,] but their formula does nothing to replace the oxidized metals which leaves the enzymes without the needed metal cofactors in order to rapidly catalyze biochemical reactions.

In Chapter 16 titled "To the Point" I detail what the seven problems are, that are involved in Alzheimer's and what needs to be done to reverse the problems.

Think about this, if you want to reverse a problem, [Alzheimer's] wouldn't you have to reverse the cause of the problem in order to succeed.

Testing methyl-eugenol, ethyl-vanillin and an emulsifier on myself, in my food and drink, I have come to the following conclusion. My age weakened immune and biochemical defense system, can no longer counter these combined chemical additives. Unless I replace the six inhibited atomic elements in my body on a regular basis.

For more information see our web site at, www.zapalzheimers. com.

The replacement therapy restores my normal memory:

These same chemical food and drink additives had been no problem for me until I reached about 65 years of age. This was about the age that memory problems also appeared in my mother, and eventually became the Alzheimer's disease that took her life.

Next, regarding Vanillin, we find more cautious news:

The following web site,

http://chemcourses.ucsd.edu/coursepages/uglabs/msds/vanillin. -Info.htm *from the University of California, S. D. Chemistry &* *Biochemistry* **states the following information regarding vanillin;**

"Toxicological information.

Section 11 acute effects.

Harmful if swallowed.

May be harmful if inhaled.

May be harmful if absorbed through the skin.

Causes eye irritation.

May cause skin irritation.

November 13, 2000, page two and three."

I wonder if, neuroresearcher Dr. Eddie Koo, of the University of California, S.D., has seen the above report. I have great respect and admiration for Dr. Eddie Koo and all of the other neuroscientists whose work I have followed for several years now.

If I were young again, I would not worry about going to the dentist. But now, my Alzheimer's research has shown me there may be an age related danger in the chemical eugenol used in his office, and also may be in prescription medicine. I am sure that dentists are not aware of this problem. Someone should tell them.

My research also raises these questions:

If I have any neuronal problems, like Alzheimer's disease [AD,] Parkinson's disease [PD,] Huntington's disease [HD] Amyotrophic Lateral Sclerosis [ALS,] or Creutzfeldt-Jakob disease [CJD] would I want methyl-eugenol, ethyl-vanillin combined with emulsifiers put in my body? "I don't think so."

If my immune system has weakened, how would these three combined chemicals affect my brain cells, including my DNA, RNA, and protein structure, mitochondria and ATP energy?

Vanillin, distilled from eugenol when combined with alcohol, ethyl-vanillin, and light [electromagnetic radiation] produces dehydrodivanillin [a product found in other solvents.] Is this causing inflammation by destroying nerve cells and tissue?

Cattle are fed vanillin worldwide. Cattle feed also contains emulsifiers, combined with vanillin.

Can there be a connection here to the mad cow disease? Bovine Spongiform Encelphalopathy [BSE.]

A study published in China, has shown that in Alzheimer's disease and Creutzfeldt Jakob disease [CJD], the human form of mad cow disease, the structure of the prion proteins is similar.

"From the BBC News titled "Alzheimer's and CJD similar." The article says, "Professor Chi Ming Yang, of University in Tiajin, China, has discovered that these proteins have very similar structures" *The article goes on to say,* "Professor Yang used a computer model to map the prion protein associated with vCJD and the amyloid precursor protein associated with early stage Alzheimer's. He found that the two proteins had a similar pattern of component parts known as amino acids." *Dr. Yang says,* "This could mean that the molecular mechanism underlying Alzheimer's disease and vCJD is the same."

More information is found on the uses of Eugenol:

The following web site,

http://www.handafc.demon.co.uk/eugenol.htm. from United States Pharmacopeia offers more information regarding eugenol, the site says, "Eugenol; usp grade, has uses in food, dental and pharmaceutical industries. Eugenol is widely used in dentistry to cover cavities, fill canals, etc."

Eugenol is toxic:

NTP Chemical Repository, Radian Corporation web site,

http://www.handafc.demon.co.uk/eugenol.htm .relates that, "August 29, 1991. Page 3 of eight, eugenol sax [surface antigen, x linked]. Toxicity evaluation.

Moderately toxic by ingestion, intraperitoneal and subcutaneous routes."

Regarding eugenol, *the National Institute of Health [NIH] web site,* *http://ntpdb.niehs.nih.gov/ntp_reports/ntp_chem_h&s/ntp_ chem9radian 97-53-0.txt May 23, 2000 relates that,* "An experimental carcinogen and tumorigen. Human mutagenic data. A human skin irritant."

Can Eugenol affect the Mitochondria?

Remember mitochondria, the producer of adenosine triphosphate [ATP,] the energy that powers brain cells?

Mitochondria defects and Alzheimer's disease:

An article published in the New York Times, USA,

Regarding Alzheimer's disease, and titled "Mitochondria defects linked to Alzheimer's disease" states, "Medical researchers at the University of Virginia Health Systems, report a direct link between abnormal mitochondria genes and amyloid proteins that cause brain cell damage, and cell death in Alzheimer's disease."

Has anyone thought about toxic eugenol and ethyl-vanillin, combined with double emulsifiers and alcohol entering the brain cell combined with amino acids, peptides, fats and proteins where it can interfere with mitochondria's work?

Eugenol and vanillin do not mix easily with water [though here, I am wondering how the emulsifiers might alter that].

Think about this. Our cells soak up water like a sponge. This explains why we can live longer without food than we can without water. Eugenol and vanillin are practically non-water soluble, so they can not enter our cells very easily. However, what happens when we add an emulsifier to this mix? An emulsifier allows water and oils to mix. Now eugenol and vanillin may enter our cells with the help of an age weakened immune system. This means they may penetrate into the center of our cells, [the nucleus] where our DNA is located. The very DNA that transcripts the genetic code for protein building to mRNA [messenger ribonucleic acid.] Are these combined chemicals [artificial flavors and emulsifiers] causing genetic mutations?

Can this be the source of the amyloid plaque found in Alzheimer's disease, or say, as an example of genetic mutation, apoe 4 the Alzheimer's gene on chromosome 19? Or on other Alzheimer genes, such as, presenilin 1 on chromosome 14, and presenilin 2 on chromosome 1, or APP gene on chromosome 21?

Medical statistics regarding Alzheimer's disease states that 5% of the cases are inherited, and 95% are sporadic.

The following web site, http://www.inchem.org/documents/sids/sids/ sids5b06.html, says, "Toxicity of vanillin to lettuce using water with 650 plus **or** minus 30 mg/1 produced a 50% reduction in germination."

Those in charge at the Institute of Toxicology, Ministry of Health, Soborg, Denmark, suspected there was a problem with ethyl-vanillin in food and drink.

The web site http://www.inchem.org/documents/jecfa/jecmono/v35je07. htm, pages, one through eight, Oct, 21, 2001, says, "Ethyl vanillin was first evaluated at the eleventh meeting of the committee [annex 1, reference 14], when an ADI [acceptable daily intake] of zero-10 mg/kg was allocated on the basis of a long-term study on rats. At the time, the committee noted that few metabolism studies had been carried out on ethyl vanillin." *The site continues, by saying,* "During the course of the next three meetings the ADI was lowered to an ADI of zero-3mg/kg for ethyl-vanillin." **That's a 70% reduction.**

In my opinion, the above information does not take into consideration that ethyl-vanillin may accumulate in an elderly persons body and may become toxic to a persons biochemical system.

Propylene-glycol and Emulsifiers:

The Kirk-Othmer Encyclopedia of Chemical Technology, 3rd Ed, Volumes 1-2, New York, NY. John Wiley and Sons, 1978-1984, V12, page 102, states that, "**Propylene glycol is present at 5-wt%, as a [solvent] in permanent hair colorant formulation for a medium brown shade.**"

The following web site http://www.lci-koeln.de/498engl.html, February 16, 2001, relates the following information regarding emulsifiers. Titled "PGPR - Small quantities, large effect" the site says, "Chemically seen is polyglycerol - polyricinoleat. [PGPR], e 476. A condensation product from polyglycerol and condensed ricinolic acids." *The site says,* "PGPR - is a highly developed emulsifying agent. PGPR - influences the yield stress more significantly and more specifically than Lecithin." *Reporting further the site says,* "Soya lecithin is also an emulsifier. The combination of both substances acts synergistically in the rheological behavior of the chocolate masses. This means that the results achieved with the optimum amount of lecithin can even be increased by adding PGPR." *The report further states,* "Because many emulsifying mechanisms are not quite clear, a research project with the title, "Relationship between texture and functional properties of emulsifiers for chocolate production at the Technical University Dresden in cooperation with the German Research Institute in Garching is being planned."

Concerning Alzheimer's disease, my findings are, adding two emulsifiers together in a product of food and drink could be like *"double trouble"* in a weakened biochemical system, especially if the emulsifiers are combined with ethyl-vanillin. This increases the effects, as is the case of PGPR combined with a second emulsifier such as soya lecithin.

Emulsifiers combined with methyl-eugenol and ethyl-vanillin did not affect my memory until I was well into my 60's. After all, this could explain why younger people with stronger biochemical systems are not having memory problems, like us older people are.

Emulsifiers allow water and oil to mix:

Concerning Emulsifiers, the on line Encyclopedia Britannica, states the following information, "Emulsifiers are used in foods of numerous chemical additives that encourage the suspension of one liquid in another, as in the mixing of oil and water in margarine, shortening, ice cream and salad dressing. Closely related to emulsifiers are stabilizers, substances that maintain the emulsified state." *Britannica also states that,* "Emulsifiers, stabilizers and related compounds are used in the preparation of cosmetics, lotions and certain pharmaceuticals, where they serve much the same purpose as in foods."

Soya lecithin is another emulsifier used. *Commenting on Lecithin the Britannica says,* "Among the products in which it is used are animal feeds, baking products and mixes, chocolate, cosmetics and soaps, dyes, insecticides, paints and plastics."

Eugenol and ethyl-vanillin. A problem for neurotransmitters?

The American Heritage, Stedman's Medical Dictionary, describes Norepinephrine as, "A substance, both a hormone and neurotransmitter, secreted by the adrenal medulla and the nerve endings of the sympathetic nervous system to cause vasoconstriction and increases in heart rate, blood pressure and the sugar level of the blood. Also called noradrenalin."

Eugenol blocks nerve transmission:

Regarding Eugenol and the Neurotransmitter Noradrenalin, the web site, *http://www.inchem.org/documents/jecfa/jecmono/v17je10htm says,* "Eugenol was reported to inhibit respiration in vitro in mitochondria isolated from the liver of adult male, Charles River rats [Cotmore et al., 1979.]" *The site continues,* "At 1 mM concentration, eugenol was reported to cause a 61% inhibition of noradrenaline induced oxidative metabolism in isolated brown fat cells from adult hamsters [Peterson et el., 1980.]" *The site further relates that,* "Eugenol is used as a dental analgesic [Tyler et al., 1977]; the compound relieves pain from irritated or diseased tooth pulp, but is not a true local anaesthetic [Stitch & Smith, 1971.]"

On page three of the report regarding Eugenol and frog tests it says, "Frog 0.1-100% direct exposure of nerve. Blockage of transmission of evoked impulses in exposed sciatic nerve, [Kozam, 1977.]"

Eugenol caused a 61% inhibition of the neurotransmitter, noradrenaline [norepinephrine?]

Eugenol blocked the nerve impulses of the neurotransmitter. [Think interruption of modulation]

Remember the old Red Cross toothache medicine? How it numbed our gums and blocked the pain. Red Cross toothache medicine contains 85% eugenol.

The web site, http://vitawise.com/clove.htm says, **"Today, clove oil, like all spice is 60-90 percent eugenol.** It is used by dentists as an oral anesthetic and to disinfect root canals." *The site says,* "Demand for clove helped launch the age of exploration. Magellan's Flotilla brought some back to Spain in 1512."

Some of these neurodegenerative diseases can also be traced back to that time. Hmmm!

The web site, http://www.pacifichealth.com/gras_list.htm. Lists emulsifying agents as,

"Cholic acid.

Desoxycholic acid.

Diacetyl tartaric acid.

Esters of mono-and diglycerides.

Glycocholic acid.

Monosodium phosphate derivatives.

Propylene glycol.
Ox bile extract.
Taurocholic acid."

The web site, http://www.pacifichealth.com/gras_list.htm. lists Stabilizers as,
"Acacia [gum Arabic.]
Agar-agar.
Ammonium alginate.
Calcium alginate.
Carob bean gum.
Chondrus extract.
Ghatti gum.
Guar gum.
Potassium alginate.
Sodium alginate.
Sterculia [or karava] gum.
Tragacanth."

When I think about propylene-glycol and ethyl-vanillin being used in the preparation of bakery products, and that propylene-glycol is used as a solvent in permanent hair coloring, anti-freeze and brake fluids, it gives me cause for concern that it is put into our foods. This may not be a problem for a young person, but I believe it may be for the elderly.

Confusing information:

It is confusing, with all the synonyms and identifiers for methyl-eugenol and ethyl-vanillin, as pointed out in Chapter 10 titled, "Exposed." When adding propylene glycol, we find it has over 13 synonyms and identifiers and can be an emulsifier.

As you read through this book, consider that when you read ethyl-vanillin on food labels, what you are reading is double to triple strength vanillin. Saying this in a different way, ethyl-vanillin is a double to triple strength oxidizer.

CHAPTER TWELVE:
MELATONIN

The Mosby Medical Encyclopedia refers to Melatonin as, "A hormone released into the blood stream by the pineal gland in the brain. When injected into a patient, melatonin causes drowsiness."

Is a lack of melatonin the reason that Alzheimer's patients have trouble sleeping? My mother, who was diagnosed with Alzheimer's disease, also had trouble sleeping at night. I have also experienced this.

Tryptophan, Melatonin, Serotonin and Niacin:

<u>Melatonin plays a major role in the bodies immune defenses against hydroxyl radicals.</u>

Neuroscience Notes says, "Melatonin is a hormone secreted by the pineal gland during night-time darkness, and is now being marketed in the U.S. as a nutritional supplement." *Continuing on, the publication says,* "The hormone is an indoleamine compound derived from the amino acid tryptophan with serotonin as an intermediate precursor."

So, we see, that tryptophan is responsible for the production of not only melatonin but also serotonin and niacin [Vitamin B-3.] Since melatonin is a major anti-oxidant, anything inhibiting melatonin production in the body or destroying the bodies store of melatonin could have major consequences on the bodies immune system, and its defenses against free radicals.

Melatonin as an antioxidant:

According to the Life Extension Foundations, web site, http://www. lef.org/prod_desc/mela01.htm, "Melatonin may be the most important anti-oxidant supplement you can take. Most anti-oxidant nutrients have difficulty penetrating cell membranes. Melatonin, on the other hand, enters cells and subcellular compartments with ease."

I am thinking about the low energy level in the Alzheimer's patient's brain. Brain cell energy comes from mitochondria's production of adinosine triphosphate [ATP] produced within the cell. I believe the two combined chemical additives [artificial flavors and emulsifiers] turned toxins, are producing free radicals, and may be interfering with the production of ATP. Melatonin has the ability to enter the cell and attack the toxin or free radical oxidants, but, if it were inhibited or destroyed, then melatonin would not be available to work this process.

Melatonin has cell access:

The Life Extension Foundation, commenting on the article, by Russell J. Retire, et. al., Department of Cellular and Structural Biology, University of Texas Health Science Center, San Antonio, Texas says, "If an antioxidant is to protect intracellular molecules from oxidative damage, the molecule providing the protection must have access to sub-cellular compartment i.e. the mitochondria and melatonin meets this requirement admirably."

Melatonin production declines with age:

The Life Extension Foundation, further relates that, "Women seem to be at risk of Alzheimer's more so than men are. It seems as we get older our body starts to lose some of its defenses." *The Foundation says,* "One consequence of aging is a declining number of melatonin-producing cells in the pineal gland and a decline in the amount of melatonin secreted by surviving melatonin producing cells. Melatonin is the primary hormonal product of the pineal gland, a photoneuroendocrine transducer and biological pacemaker that affects the seasonal adaptation of higher animals governs a variety of reproductive and immunoregulatory functions and may play a role in cancer, aging and senescence [the state of being old.]"

Regarding Melatonin and Oxidation:

Titled, "Melatonin and its Function as an Anti-oxidant," by Desi Kreska, 2425 Organic Chemistry, Ralph Logan-Instructor, April 16, 1997, says, "Melatonin is said to be the best anti-oxidant according to R. J. Reiter author of the book on the subject. It is 500 times more effective on free radicals than DMSO."

Continuing on, Kreska says, "Directly and indirectly melatonin is said to exert a powerful anti-oxidant effect, which is metabolized in all body tissue. Some reports say that melatonin is the most powerful anti-oxidant of all."

Melatonin extends life in older mice:

The Life Extension Foundation, reports that, "Not only does melatonin production decline clinically with age, but administration of melatonin or the implantation of pineal tissue from young donors prolongs both median and absolute survival times of older mice" *states Dr. Leland N. Edmunds, Jr. Division of Biological Sciences, State University of New York, Stonybrook, New York.*

I think these three combined chemical additives, I have isolated, are helping to cause my Alzheimer's disease, by inhibiting the production of melatonin in my body.

Does ethyl-vanillin combined with emulsifiers, in an aged body, cause melatonin reduction?

A recent newspaper article regarding calories and fat in the diet, titled, "High Fats, Calories May Boost Alzheimer's Risk for Some." *Lindsey Tanner, AP Medical Writer, Chicago, reported that,* "A diet high in calories and fat may increase the risk of Alzheimer's disease in people who are genetically susceptible to the mind-robbing disorder, new research suggests." *Tanner says,* "The study found that people who consumed the most calories and fat faced double the risk of developing Alzheimer's." *Lead author of the study, Dr. Jose Luchsinger, is an Alzheimer's researcher at Columbia University.*

Testing on myself, over a three year plus time frame, my findings are, it is <u>not calories and fats</u> that caused my cognitive impairment. It just happens that calories and fats are in the same areas of food and drink that contain the methyl-eugenol and ethyl-vanillin [artificial flavors] and emulsifiers.

Let's use common logic. If we were to go on a diet to reduce calories what foods would we want to stay away from? Candies, soft drinks, bakery products, donuts, pies, rolls, cakes with icings and ice creams. These are the very products that contain the methyl-eugenol, ethyl-vanillin [artificial flavors] combined with double emulsifier additives that I have found to be causing my Alzheimer's symptoms, when combined with an age weakened immune and biochemical system.

In my mind, this recent study regarding calories and fats only reinforces my findings, that these combined chemical additives become a problem only when the immune system or the biochemical system weakens from aging.

It should be obvious to anyone reading this, that, calories and fats just happen to be in the same food and drink that also contain these combined chemical additives.

In a report by The Life Extension Foundation, titled, "Melatonin Increases during Calorie Restriction," The Foundation says, "Calorie restriction consistently produce radical increases in lifespan and reduction of cancers in animal studies." Reporting further, Dr. Gerald Huethers, researcher at Psychiatrische Universitasklinik, Gottingen, Germany, says, "New studies show that calorie restriction causes an increase in serum melatonin and scientists are speculating that this may be one of the reasons why severe calorie restriction extends lifespan so dramatically."

"Melatonin increases during calorie restriction?"

In my opinion, I see it differently. I would say,

"Melatonin increases as the combined chemical food and drink additives decreases."

Reducing calorie intake also reduces the intake of methyl-eugenol, ethyl-vanillin [artificial flavors] and emulsifiers. According to my findings, these combined chemical food and drink additives are at the heart of the problem with my Alzheimer's disease. Anyone not having memory problems may not notice any cognitive impairment from these chemicals until they are older. In my opinion, this is one reason it has been so difficult to unlock the mystery of the Alzheimer's disease.

The words I watch for on packages are vanillin, ethyl-vanillin [artificial flavors,] emulsifier and vanilla extract. In vanilla extract, I will get both alcohol and vanillin.

When reading the following, keep in mind my earlier question regarding where these chemical additives eugenol, vanillin, alcohol and emulsifiers go, that are combined in food and drink when we ingest them?

The Life Extension Foundation, website reports that, "A new study also confirms that melatonin is synthesized in parts of the body other than just the pineal gland. The retina in the eye, which is exposed to continuous ultraviolet oxidative damage, is the most acknowledged independent site of melatonin synthesis in vertebrates." Melatonin produced in the retina? Comes to mind that vanillin, mixed with alcohol, and exposed to light, [the retina receives light] converts to dehydrodivanillin, a product found in other solvents. [Solvents are to dissolve, in this case, maybe melatonin.] *Reporting further on Dr. Huether's work, the site says,* "In this study, melatonin was found to be more abundantly produced in the gastrointestinal tract than even the pineal gland. Site of the melatonin synthesis, the enterochromaffin cells of the gastrointestinal tract."

Amyloid plaque has been found in the cataracts of Alzheimer's patients.

I believe these three combined chemicals may be destroying melatonin in the gastrointestinal tract, thereby, disarming the immune system. <u>In an aged body, are the chemicals methyl-eugenol and ethyl-vanillin [artificial flavors,] when combined with an emulsifier becoming toxic and causing the immune system to attack itself?</u>

Can these combined chemicals also be causing DNA mutation?

The web site,
http://www.lef.org/prod_desc/mela01.htm reports that,
"Numerous synthetic and natural compounds mutate cellular DNA, and cause cancer cells to form. Aging cells lose their DNA gene repair mechanisms and the result is that DNA genetic damage can cause cells to proliferate out of control, i.e., and turn into cancer cells."

Melatonin and Zinc restore immune function:

The web site, http://www.lef.org/prod_desc/mela01.htm , reports on the research of Dr. Eugenio Mocchegiani, Immunology Center, Italian National Research Centers on Aging that, "Zinc absorption is strongly reduced in the elderly, sometimes even in those who take supplemental nutrients. Melatonin supplementation enables older animals that are zinc deficient to absorb and use zinc more effectively."

If you have an interest in Alzheimer's, cancer or aging, I recommend all of the sources I have reviewed in this book.

In Alzheimer's patients, zinc supplements can inhibit folic acid, causing a cascade of problems. *Regarding chronic inflammation, The Life Extension Foundation, says,* "Aging people suffer an epidemic of outward inflammatory diseases such as arthritis, but chronic inflammation also damages brain cells, arterial walls, heart valves and other structures in the body. Heart attack, stroke, heart valve failure, and Alzheimer's senility has been linked to the chronic inflammatory cascade so often seen in aging humans."

Do these combined chemical additives have the ability to alter DNA? Could this explain the mutation of the familial Alzheimer's gene, apoe4 that can be inherited from parents?

When these chemical additives are combined, and the age related immune system is weakened, couldn't this set the stage to render the *"six elements,"* electrically static and non functional, thereby, needing to replace them on a continual basis?

Could this also be the path that manifests electrically static Cancer cells?

CHAPTER THIRTEEN:
ALUMINUM

One piece of this puzzle is aluminum.

The web site, www.merriam-webster.com, describes Aluminum as, "A bluish silver-white malleable ductile light trivalent metallic element that has good electrical and thermal conductivity, high reflectivity and resistance to oxidation and is the most abundant metal in the earth's crust, where it always occurs in combination."

I believe the process that produces Alzheimer's dementia is a very complicated one. The logical is obvious. Many highly educated researchers are being left at the gate in this race for answers.

The problem with Aluminum cookware:

The web site, www.connectcorp.net/~trufax/mercury/alum1.html says, "Along with aluminum foil, cookware made of aluminum is a significant source of excess aluminum in the diet. Boiling water in aluminum containers, especially water containing acidic substances, causes aluminum to leach into the water and food." *The site continues on to say,* "Water containing fluorides encourages the leaching process from aluminum cookware." *Continuing on, the web site says,* "An article in Nature Magazine, on, January 15, 1987, revealed that,* when cooking, if fluoridated water is used with aluminum cookware, the aluminum more readily leaches from the cookware into the food."

The following web site, http://www.futuredynamicadvantage.com/trufax/fluoride/aluminum.html, states the following information titled, "Aluminum and fluoride: synergistic action." *The site says,* "There is aluminum in the water in the form of aluminum sulfate [alum] that is deliberately added to precipitate solid waste matter at the water treatment plant. Aluminum would ordinarily break down into aluminum oxide and weak sulfuric acid, which would not be a problem as aluminum oxide would simply pass through the digestive system. The weak sulfuric acid would be diluted to the point of insignificance." *The web site relates the following information,* "The picture changes radically, relative to the breakdown of aluminum sulfate, when fluorides are added to the public water supply, the aluminum sulfate becomes aluminum fluoride and weak sulfuric acid." *Continuing on the site says,* "Aluminum fluoride is acted on by the hydrochloric acid in the stomach, allowing the aluminum oxide to be deposited inside the organs and brain instead of being passed through."

Titled, *"The Neurological and Physiological Effect of Aluminum Deposition" the web site, http://www.connectcorp.net/~trufax/mercury/alum.html, says,* "Aluminum is known to be a significant cross-linking agent that acts to immobilize reactive molecules within brain cells." We have all heard a lot about free radicals. *Regarding aluminum, the web site states,* "It also causes free radical pathology inside the neurons, bringing on molecular cross-linkage throughout the brain's tissues, resulting in neurofibrillary tangles so characteristic of those seen in autopsies of brains of those with Alzheimer's syndrome."

Mother stopped cooking with aluminum pans, but, of course, the disease was already manifested.

The web site,

http://www.futuredynamicadvantage.com/trufax/fluoride/aluminum.html, says, "Consider the fact that when you have diet beverages in cans, you have the following cocktail: Fluoridated water-free fluoride ions, phosphoric or citric acids, which allow the aluminum ions to break down from the can." *Continuing, on the site says,* "Aluminum ions from the can, allow the fluorides too more easily, pass the blood-brain barrier. Aluminum fluoride forms the combination of fluorine and aluminum ions. Sugar, which also allows the fluorides too more easily pass the blood-brain barrier."

Regarding aspartame, the site says, "Aspartame, which caused neurological damage in league with the fluorides. If the cans are stored above 80 degrees, the aspartame breaks down into carcinogenic formaldehyde and toxic methanol. Of course, it is also over 80 degrees inside the body. The methanol also affects the brain."

<u>The methanol also affects the brain?</u>
[Methanol is alcohol]

"Be careful of your thoughts, they may
become words at any moment."
Ira Gassen.

Propylene-glycol and ethyl-vanillin!

CHAPTER FOURTEEN:
CALORIES, DIET
AND
THE TEST

There are several studies out there that imply, calories are implicated in Alzheimer's disease. Is it really the calories? Or, is it, that the calories just happen to be in the same areas of certain food and drinks which also contains methyl-eugenol and ethyl-vanillin [artificial flavors], combined with emulsifiers like propylene glycol and soya lecithin?

An article in the newspaper, Houston Chronicle, titled, "Mediterranean Diet May Cut Alzheimer's Risk," backs my hypothesis, that certain combined chemical additives in our food and drinks are causing not only Alzheimer's disease, but also heart disease.

The article written by Malcolm Ritter of the Associated Press, states that, "People who followed the diet were up to 40 percent less likely, than those who largely avoided it, to develop Alzheimer's during the course of the research, scientists reported."

Reporting further, the article says, "Dr. Nikolaos Scarmeas, of the Columbia University Medical Center here, [New York] lead author of the research said, "Still more research must be done before the diet can be recommended to ward off Alzheimer's."

Continuing on the article says, "Previous research has suggested that such an approach can cut the risk of heart disease." *In the article, Dr. Marilyn Albert, a Johns Hopkins Neurology professor and spokeswoman for the Alzheimer's Association, said,* "The idea that a heart-healthy diet could also help fight Alzheimer's, fits in with growing evidence that the kinds of things that we associate with being bad for our heart turn out to be bad for our brain."

My findings are, that the oxidizers [methyl-eugenol and ethyl-vanillin] combined with double strength emulsifiers may be the culprits that are causing Alzheimer's disease and heart disease.

I also believe, the reason a Mediterranean diet is beneficial is, because, it does not contain these chemical food and drink additives, [artificial flavors and emulsifiers.] These foods contain the elements that replace the *"six atomic elements"* that have been inhibited.

Let's review another one of these studies. *Published in the AARP Bulletin dated, September 2002, titled: "How to Reduce Your Risk for Alzheimer's," the article says,* "Don't get to big, eat a healthy diet and stay active, physically and mentally," *William Thies, Vice President of the Alzheimer's Association said at July's International conference on Alzheimer's disease in Stockholm.*

Reporting on other news from the meeting the report says, "Researchers recommend a low fat diet with five servings of fruits and vegetables a day, fish, and vitamin-B and vitamin-C."

Guess what the above foods contain? Trace elements and minerals, the *"six numbers"* [the six elements]

Researchers at Case Western University, School of Medicine and University Hospitals of Cleveland, Ohio, found that, "A diet of more fruit and vegetables and less red meat offers more protection against the development of Alzheimer's." [that red meat when on the hoof, are fed vanillin and emulsifiers.]

Here again, fruits and vegetables contain the six trace elements, vitamins and minerals.

BBC News, dated July 21, 2002, reports that, "Having a healthy diet, exercising and not being overweight can not only reduce the risk of developing heart disease, but may also protect against Alzheimer's, new research claims." I believe that's true.

The news report goes on to say, "So far, doctors have been unsure about what causes Alzheimer's disease, however, both genetic and environmental influences are thought to play a part." *Continuing on the report says,* "Scientists still do not know exactly why and how the disease develops, but, the biggest risk is simply age. Alzheimer's cases double with every five years of age between 65 and 85." The article goes on to speak about vitamins.

This is a good time to bring up a point. We hear about vitamins constantly and rightly so. They are not only very important to our health, but they also act as co-factors with the enzymes in our body.

Here is the point. When was the last time someone told us how important trace mineral elements are to our bodies? It seems the total focus has been only on vitamins.

The following web site, http://www.anyvitamins.com/trace-elements-info.htm, says, "Trace elements are also known as micronutrients and are found only in minute quantities in the body-yet they are vitally important. The quantities in which they are found are so small that they can only be detected by spectrographic methods or by using radioactive elements." *The web site further states that,* "The interaction of these micronutrients are difficult to study, since they are found occurring together in various forms and amounts in the diet, and their absorption from the intestinal tract may be dependent on their relative concentrations, and might be synergetic or antagonistic, and the amount could depend on the amount of other essential trace elements in the diet."

The article on the web site says, "The following are considered essential micronutrients: cobalt, copper, chromium, fluorine, iron, iodine, manganese, molybdenum, selenium and zinc."

The article further relates that, "On the other hand, nickel, tin, vanadium, silicon and boron have recently been found as important micronutrients, whereas aluminum, arsenic, barium, bismuth, bromine, cadminum, germanium, gold, lead, lithium, mercury, rubidium, silver, strontium, titanium and zirconium, is all found in plant and animal tissue, yet their importance is still being determined."

The above article mentions fluorine [atomic number 9,] iron [atomic number 26,] silicon [atomic number 14] and lithium [atomic number 3.] This identifies four of the six numbers [elements] and how important they are to our health.

The other two not mentioned are nitrogen [atomic number 7] and sodium [atomic number 11.] Life could not exist without nitrogen, and sodium.

Trace Minerals Research [Concentrace] web site, http://www.traceminerals.com/ions.html, states, "Like your body, it only lights up with ionic trace minerals. Every second of every day your body relies on ionic minerals and trace elements to conduct and generate billions of tiny electrical impulses." *The site goes on to say,* "Without these impulses, not a single muscle, including your heart, would be able to function. Your brain would not function and the cells would not be able to use osmosis to balance water pressure and absorb nutrients." *The article goes on to say,*

"Whatever the nutritional potential of a food, its contribution is nonexistent if it does not pass the test of absorption. Those minerals that your body is unable to break down to their ionic form are likely to pass completely from the body unassimilated, and for all nutritional intents and purposes, were never eaten."

Is the absorption of nutrients, through osmosis, being inhibited by double emulsifiers that confuse water and fats, by mixing together?

In the above article, authors Dr. Rosenburg and Dr. Solomons offer the following insight, "Minerals that are absorbed in their ionic form are in true liquid solution and have either positive or negative charges. They also have unique properties that distinguish them from each other and allow them to freely take part in biochemical communication throughout the body." The authors continue by saying that, "These communications help nutrients move to those areas of the body that are in most need of their help." *According to Rosenburg and Solomons,* "Imbalances of any of these ions or certain trace ions in the body can lead to dysfunction in the conduction of electrical messages. This dysfunction quickly leads to a general body disturbance and loss of ability to maintain somewhat stable internal conditions."

An article reported in the newspaper, Houston Chronicle, Tuesday, July 15, 2003, by Deanna Bellandi, Associated Press Chicago, says, "A study found that overweight women may have a higher risk of developing Alzheimer's. " *Lead author of the study, Deborah Gustafson, said,* "I think that what it means is that overweight and obesity continue to be a public health problem and that as women age it's still something that women need to be concerned about in relationship to their health risks."

After reading the above information, the things that come to my mind are, there is more involved here than calories and obesity. I think the Alzheimer's risk is not about calories, but is about the combined chemical food and drink additivies methyl-eugenol and ethyl-vanillin [artificial flavors] combined with double emulsifiers. I believe, that all artificial flavors including vanillin, are a threat to my memory, because, my immune system and biochemical defense system has weakened from aging.

There has been a lot of information lately concerning obesity and fast food establishments. I want to share with you some of my research findings. These are the things I found that increased my memory problems.

The following are some of the desserts sold at fast food establishments and the chemicals they contain:

Birthday cake yellow:
Vanillin [artifical flavor]
Mono and diglycerides [emulsifiers]
Birthday cake chocolate:
Vanillin [artificial flavor]
Mono and diglycerides [emulsifiers]
Chocolate chip cookies:
Artificial flavors
Vanilla flavored shake syrup:
Propylene glycol [emulsifier]
Ethyl vanillin [alcohol and artifical flavor]
Vanillin [artificial flavor]

Strawberry flavored shake syrup:
Propylene glycol [emulsifier]
Artificial flavors
Shake mix:
Guar gum [emulsifier]
Imitation vanilla [artificial flavor]
Oreo cookie pieces:
Soy lechithin [emulsifier]
Vanillin [artificial flavor]
Nestle Crunch:
Soy lecithin [emulsifier]
Vanillin [artifical flavor]

M&M pieces:
Soy lecithin [emulsifier]

Artificial flavors

Lowfat yogurt:
Artificial flavors
Butterfinger pieces:
Soy lecithin [emulsifier]
Monoglycerides [emulsifier]
Artificial flavors

Cone:

Vanillin [artificial flavor]

Hot carmel topping:
Ethyl vanillin [alcohol and artificial flavor]
Vanillin [artificial flavor]
Hot fudge topping:
Vanillin [artificial flavor]
Strawberry topping:
Artificial flavors
Vanilla reduced fat ice cream:
Mono and diglycerides [emulsifiers]
Guar gum [emulsifier]
Vanilla [artificial flavor]

All the above products make us fat. The products from bakeries also contain these same chemicals, as do many candies. It is not calories that causes Alzheimer's according to my findings. It is methyl-eugenol and ethyl-vanillin [artificial flavors] and emulsifiers in combination. However, a young immune system is protective.

Have you ever seen a teenager with Alzheimer's?

The following information by Reuters-Health Wednesday, August 14, 5:36 PM ET 2002, says, "High-calorie diets loaded with fats may spell trouble for people with a genetic predisposition for the memory-robbing Alzheimer's disease, the results of a new study suggests." *Investigators at Columbia University in New York City reports that,* "People with apolipoprotein E e-4 [Apo e-4] a genetic variant linked with Alzheimer's disease who consume the most calories and fat are twice as likely to develop Alzheimer's compared with those consuming the least amount. Bottom line, they conclude that the current findings suggest the possibility of modifying the risk of Alzheimer's disease with caloric restriction and low-fat diets in susceptible individuals."

When calories are restricted, methyl-eugenol and ethyl-vanillin [artificial flavors] and emulsifiers [solvents] are also restricted, aren't they?

There are millions of heart breaking stories regarding this Alzheimer's disease. The following web site in the next paragraph, relates one such story.

The web site,

<u>*http://members.nbci.com/ XMCM/sexylegz/alzheimers.*</u>

<u>*Html,*</u> *dated February 11, 2001, says,* "Caring for two disabled parents hasn't been easy for this family, but, it's their way of giving back to the couple who raised them. It's our turn. Elizabeth always had been a candy lover, but when she began hoarding it, her family knew it was yet another symptom of what they had come to deal with. The Alzheimer's disease that was slowly debilitating their mother. " *The web site says,* "Elizabeth sometimes loaded three grocery carts full of Snickers bars. She hoarded other items too, buying 50 light bulbs at a time."

Continuing on the web site says, "We probably found 150-200 snickers all throughout her socks and stuffed between the mattress and the box springs, tucked away in the curtains." *Elizabeth's daughter Mary says* "She had snickers bars and M&M's everywhere. Elizabeth, 68, once loved to go to rummage sales and buy dolls.

She liked to make homemade meals, bake apple pies and cinnamon rolls and to can tomatoes. Elizabeth's husband Robert suffered a disabling stroke." *Story by Tamara Browning.*

So many sad stories concerning this Alzheimer's disease.

Some candy bars contain the following:

Snickers candy bars contains:
Artificial flavors
Emulsifiers

M&M candy contains:
Artificial flavors
Emulsifiers

Apple pies contain:
Vanilla extract [alcohol]
Vanillin [artificial flavor]

Cinnamon rolls contain:
Artificial flavors
Emulsifiers

I have eaten these same products and other candies all my life with no problems, until I reached 65 years of age. At that age, I started having memory problems which developed from eating candies and desserts that combined the chemicals methyl-eugenol, ethyl-vanillin [artificial flavors] and emulsifiers.

Using the "*Element Replacement* " on a regular basis, I can again eat these desserts with no memory problems, although, I have cut back on them some. **For more information, see our web site at, www. zapalzheimers.com.**

In Tom Warren's fine book titled, *Beating Alzheimer's,* I think you will find evidence that supports my claim. Mr. Warren devotes 33 pages in his book to support his claim that mercury caused his Alzheimer's disease, which he was eventually able to reverse. On pages 14 and 15 of his book, he presents photos of x-rays that show the reversal of the disease.

I am sure Mercury is not good for our health. **What I want to point out here is something Mr. Warren causally wrote .** *On page 65, of his book, Mr Warren states,* "I have been taking Trace Mineral Supplements for several years now as suggested in *Orthomolecular Medicine for Physicans."* My point is, **I believe replacing the six elements contained in the Trace Mineral Supplements** Lithium [3,] Nitrogen [7,] Fluorine/Fluoride [9,] Sodium [11,] Silicon [14] and Iron [26] is responsible for reversing Mr. Warrens Alzheimer's. Not just removal of the mercury.

Tom Warren definitly had Alzheimer's, the x-rays show the amyloid plaque in his brain. Later, other x-rays showed that it was gone. The question is...what removed it?

I believe the element replacement [he states on page 65 he has been taking trace minerals for several years now] is what removed the amyloid plaque from his brain.

Here is why I do not believe mercury caused his Alzheimer's dementia. The Alzheimer's Association fact sheet says that in 1991 the Food and Drug Administration [FDA] reviewed mercury in case reports and found no evidence that amalgam poses any danger of Alzheimer's.

Also in 1991, The National Institute of Health [NIH] funded a study at the University of Kentucky and found no correlation between Alzheimer's disease and levels of mercury.

I believe it was the Element Replacement and not, the removal of mercury that reversed Tom Warrens Alzheimer's disease.

The thing I find encouring here is, after Tom Warren published his book, the powers that be, looked into it. Let's hope after publication of my book the people in charge of our health care will also evaluate my work by iniating some clinical trials. I'm betting they will find my information correct. The elderly brain can no longer tolerate strong artificial flavors combined with double and or triple emulsifiers.

When a person takes Trace Mineral Supplements they are getting the six atomic elements, and that is what restored my memory and removed the cognitive impairment.

Over a three year period of testing on myself, I have alternated back and forth between using the *"six elements"* for months and restoring my memory, then not using the *"six elements."* All the while continuing to ingest the combined chemical compound food and drink additives methyl-eugenol and ethyl-vanillin [artificial flavors] combined with emulsifiers.

It takes about 30 days of **not** replacing the "*six elements*" for small memory problems to show up. By the end of 60 days, the memory problems are, much more pronounced. By this time, some of the *six trace elements* and minerals [lithium, nitrogen, fluorine, sodium, silicon and iron,] have lost their ionic function and have been oxidized and rendered electrically static by the combined chemicals.

When I **increased** my intake of these chemicals, at this point, my memory problems accelerated and mental cognition declined rapidly. I have been able to descend deep into the Alzheimer's world several times, and I can tell you, it's a very scary experience. I choose not to go back in there again.

Here is what I use to protect myself and maintain normal cognition. I take vitamin-A, vitamin-C and vitamin-E. These vitamins reduce free radicals. I also take multiple vitamin-B tablets. I believe my main defense against Alzheimer's deficiency comes from the *"Element Replacement Therapy."* I take two or three tablets a day of Trace Mineral Supplements. One with each meal. If my will power is low and I can't resist eating some desserts which contain the artificial flavors combined with emulsifiers, then I will take one or two extra tablets of Trace Mineral Supplements.

Bottom line: I try not to eat very many desserts, unless they are made with natural flavors. This also includes jellies.

Here is proof in the pudding [is that a pun?] If I have enough will power, to not put any of the artificial flavors, combined with double emulsifiers, into my body [which is next to impossible because, this stuff is so abundant] I have found if I can do this, then the 6 elements are not being inhibited, so I can maintain normal cognition without having to replace them. This tells me, a controlled diet is imperative for an elderly person who has a loss of memory and cognitive impairment.

A word of caution! Not all trace elements contain lithium, nitrogen, fluorine [fluoride,] sodium, silicon and iron. I searched for several months, and finally settled on one brand of trace minerals. I have been using these successfully for four years now.

More information on this can be found on our website at, www. zapalzheimers.com.

THE TEST

There is a very easy way for you to test this. If you are caring for a loved one who has the early stages of Alzheimer's, simply give them some of their favorite desserts containing vanillin, artificial flavors and emulsifiers a couple of evenings in a row. Pay close attention to their cognition the next day or two. Vanilla ice cream containing vanillin [artificial flavors], vanilla extract and emulsifiers. This is one example that will do it. [only those with memory problems should be effected by this.] The cheaper the brand of ice cream, the more the memory will decline in an elderly person over age 65 or 70.

I think what you will find is their confusion and cognitive decline will be temporarily increased. I think, you will also find if they continue to ingest these combined chemicals, their mental cognition may continue to deteriorate.

If you find that what I claim is correct, I would encourage you to discuss *"Element Replacement"* with your family physican or the doctor in charge. Please, do this before your loved one reaches the third phase of Alzheimer's, where the brain cells start to degenerate and die. If you have a loved one, who has been placed in a care facility, don't give up hope. I have both pro and con research in my files

from neuroscientists regarding neurogenesis [formation of new nerve tissue.]

If my mother was still alive, and living at the Alzheimer's care facility and with the doctors approval, I would go there two or three times a day to provide her with the *"Element Replacement,"* using *trace mineral tablets.* [trace mineral liquid is also available.] I would also ask that all desserts containing artificial flavors combined with double emulsifiers be removed from her diet. Based on my experience of self testing, I would expect her **to start regaining** normal cognition within 60 to 90 days. Remember, Trace Mineral Supplements are approved safe for over the counter sales. No prescription is needed to purchase them.

See our web site at www.zapalzheimers.com for more information.

Based on my findings, if the medical profession is going to be successful in reversing Alzheimer's, they will need to expand their therapy tools. At the present time, they are trying to cure Alzheimer's by treating individual mechanisms. Years of Alzheimer's research and testing on myself has shown me that Alzheimer's is a disease of element and vitamin deficiency.

Think about it, our bodies come from the earth and our bodies contain some of the same elements that are in the earth. **It only makes sense that, if some of these elements are not functioning properly, then they need to be replaced.**

Maybe someone in the pharmaceutical industry

Will come forward and produce a therapeutic drug for us that contain the atomic element fluorine [number 9] along with the other 5 elements, lithium, nitrogen, sodium, silicon and iron.

I have a patent pending on these 6 elements.

CHAPTER FIFTEEN:
"SIX NUMBERS"
"3 – 7 – 9 – 11 – 14 – 26"

Let's examine the "*six numbers.*"
If we convert these "six numbers" *to six atomic elements from the* "Periodic Table of Elements," *we come up with the following:*
Number 03 ...Lithium
Number 07 ...Nitrogen
Number 09 ...Fluorine
Number 11 ...Sodium
Number 14 ...Silicon
Number 26 ...Iron
Now, let's examine these *"six elements"* in order to gain a better understanding of them.

Here is the first number.
Number 3 Lithium [Li]

Merriam-Webster's Collegiate Dictionary, describes Lithium, as, "A soft silver-white element of the alkali metal group that is the lightest metal known and that is used in chemical synthesis and storage batteries. A salt of lithium [as lithium carbonate] used in psychiatric medicine."

The Mineral Information Institute says, "Lithium was discovered by Johan Arfvedson, of Sweden in 1817."

The book titled, *"Total Nutrition," from The Mount Sinai School of Medicine, says,* "Lithium is used to treat manic-depression and other mood disorders, and may also promote appetite and weight gain." I have found this to be an excellent reference book.

Biochemical elements have different biological functions. Consider the following information regarding lithium and how our brain cells are designed. It speaks of the sodium channel which opens to allow ionic chemicals to enter the brain cell and depolarize it, allowing action potential.

Lithium ions:

According to Scientific American Inc, "This chemical process of action potential is necessary for us to have the ability to think. The ionic selectivity of the sodium channel partly depends on steric factors." [Author: Steric, is relating to or involving the arrangement of atoms in space.] The article continues by saying, "Na+ [positive charged sodium ions] and Li+ [positive charged lithium ions] together with a water molecule, fit in the channel, as do hydroxylamine and hydrazine." *The article continues,* "In contrast, k+ [positive charged potassium ions] with a water molecule is too large to fit in the sodium channel."

Ionic Electric Signals:

Dr. Lubert Stryer, Biochemistry, Stanford University, relates that, "Nerve impulses are electrical signals produced by the flow of ions across the plasma membrane of neurons."

Simply put, what we are looking for here is a reason to assume number 3, lithium, has a role to play in the brain. Where Alzheimer's dementia is terminating action potential, synaptic transmission, and causing cognitive impairment.

It makes logical sense to me, that if biochemistry books use lithium to describe how Na+ and Li+ combined with H_2O [water] will fit in the sodium channel, but, K+ and H_2O will not. This tells me lithium, is an important player in the function of the biochemical thought process.

While thinking about lithium and the purpose for this element in the brain, and knowing of the anger and frustration displayed by Alzheimer's patients, I find the following very interesting.

Lithium and Aggressive Behavior:

According to Burton Goldberg, in his book titled, "Studies in Alternative Medicine," he states, "Texas has shown that when levels of the trace element lithium are restored to normal levels by careful supplementation, aggressive behavior drops significantly."

An excellent book for research.

According to the Columbia Encyclopedia, "Lithium is used in the synthesis of vitamin A."

Lithium – Bcl-levels and Apoptosis:
Apoptosis is programmed cell death.

The web site, http://biopsychiatry.com/lithprot.html, says, "To date, lithium remains the only medication demonstrated to markedly increase Bcl-levels in several brain areas; in the absence of other adequate treatments, the potential efficacy of lithium, in the long term treatment of certain neurodegenerative disorders may be warranted." [Author-Bcl is a group of proteins that can initiate or inhibit cell death.]

Is protein misfolding inhibiting Bcl-2 function? "Think oxidative stress." If replacing lithium can inhibit cell death, one must ask this question: What is wrong with the lithium we get from our diet? Is the lithium ion in our diet being oxidized or mutated by double and triple strength eugenol and or ethyl-vanillin? What about double emulsifiers that also wind up in our gastrointestinal track? Do these extra strong oxidizers and emulsifiers then subdue our age-weakened immune and biochemical defense system, causing cognitive impairment?

The web site, http://www.parkinsons-information-exchange-network-online.com/drugdb/073.html, states, "Lithium is a monovalent cation similar to sodium and potassium." *Continuing on, the site relates that,* "Mechanism of action; Lithium competes at cellular sites with sodium, potassium, calcium and magnesium ions. At the cell membrane, it readily passes through sodium channels and high concentrations can block potassium channels. Lithium competes with these ions at intracellular binding sites, at protein surfaces, at carrier binding sites, and at transport sites."

Figure the odds:

Let's look at the facts here. There are 114 known atomic elements in the *"Periodic Table of Elements."* Number 3, lithium, just happens to be involved in the chemical process of thought. Figure the odds.

Here is the second number.
Number 7 Nitrogen [N]

Webster's Dictionary, describes Nitrogen, as, "A colorless tasteless odorless element that as a diatomic gas is relatively inert and constitutes 78 percent of the atmosphere by volume and that occurs as a constituent of all living tissues."

Nitrogen DNA and Proteins:

According to the Mineral Information Institute,

"Nitrogen is an important constituent of DNA nucleic acids and proteins. Nitrogen is also essential to plant and animal life and was discovered by Daniel Rutherford, of Scotland, in 1772."

Nitrogen and Vanillin:

Nitrogen in the body is blended into protein. When vanillin is exposed to protein, it loses its flavor. I believe the vanillin may be affecting the nitrogen in the protein, causing negative nitrogen balance, thereby, producing inflammation. Vanillin is an oxidizer.

How important is number 7... Nitrogen?

The Britannica.com states that, "Nitrogen is found in the nucleus of every living cell as one of the chemical components of DNA."

The web site, http://pearl1.lanl.gov/periodic/elements/7.html, says,
"The nitrogen cycle is one of the most important processes in nature for living organisms."

No doubt about it, number 7 nitrogen, is so important that life could not exist without it.

Number 7 nitrogen, is one of the *"six elements,"* I believe needs to be replaced in patients with Alzheimer's disease.

Here is the third number.
Number 9 Fluorine [F]

The web site,

http://pearl1.lanl.gov/periodic/elements/7.html, says,

"The element Fluorine was discovered in 1529, but only isolated in 1866 by Mossian in Russia." *The site further says,* "It took seventy-four years of effort and experiments to turn out successful."

Fluorine - Electronegative and Very Reactive:

The web site, http://library.thinkquest.org/co113863/fluorine.shtml states, "Fluorine is the most reactive element of all of the elements. It is also electronegative."

The web site, http://pearll.lanl.gov/periodic/elements/9.html states, "The presence of fluorine as a soluble fluoride in drinking water to the extent of 2 ppm may cause mottled enamel in teeth, when used by children acquiring permanent teeth, in smaller amounts however, fluorides are added to water supplies to prevent dental cavities." *The site also relates that,* "The recommended maximum allowable concentration for a daily 8-hour time weighted exposure is 1 ppm." [Parts per million.]

Fluorine – A Trace Element:

The web site, http://www.anyvitamins.com/fluorine-info.htm,

says, "Fluorine is a constituent of bones and teeth. In the case of microelements, such as trace elements, the amounts are very small, yet they are still important."

The web site, http://www.traceminerals.com/about.html says,

"The total trace elements in our bodies would barley fill a thimble, but that thimble full is needed to sustain life." *The site further relates that,* "Trace minerals, through biochemical communication, send nutrients to parts of the body that are most in need of help."

Acetylcholine and Trace Elements:

Without nutrients that trace minerals send, the body suffers malnutrition and the brain is unable to manufacture choline for the acetylcholine neurotransmitter. Just to name two problems caused by a deficient amount of trace minerals in our bodies.

I believe fluorine/fluoride may need to be replaced on a continual basis in Alzheimer's patients. As maybe the other five elements also. Because the *"six elements,"* are being inhibited by the double and triple strength oxidizers, eugenol, methyl-eugenol and ethyl-vanillin [artificial flavors] combined with strong emulsifiers especially propylene-glycol.

I believe, 92% of the population has no memory problems from these combined chemical food additives, at least, not until we get old and our immune and biochemical systems starts to weaken.

Here is the fourth number. Number 11 Sodium [Na]

Webster's Dictionary, describes Sodium as, "A silver white soft waxy ductile element of the alkali metal group that occurs abundantly in nature in combined form and is very active chemically."

Sodium Deficiency and Alzheimer's:

This is an easy one. Without sodium, the cells in our body would not function. The sodium-potassium pump that moves the biochemical exchanges of ions in and out of cells is necessary for us to be able to think.

The web site, http://pearl1.lanl.gov/periodic/elements/ll.html, says, "Long recognized in compounds, sodium was first isolated by Davy in 1807, by electrolysis of caustic soda." *The site further says,* "Sodium is present in fair abundance in the sun and stars. Sodium is the fourth most abundant element on earth."

There is no official RDA, [recommended daily allowance,] but *the National Academy of Science, estimates that,* "A safe daily allowance of sodium would be 500mg. for most adults." *The site says,* "Deficiency symptoms include: Decreased appetite, decreased weight, nausea, muscle weakness/cramps/ shrinkage/ blood vessel collapse, headaches, anxiety, confusion, dizziness, salt cravings, hay fever, watery eyes, runny nose, low fevers, edema, depression and deterioration of gallbladder." *It further relates that,* "Toxicity symptoms include; increased blood pressure, decreased potassium levels and coma."

Other estimates put the maximum sodium intake per day at 2400 Mg.

Here is the fifth number.
Number 14 Silicon [Si]

Webster's Dictionary, describes Silicon as, "A tetravalent nonmetallic element that occurs combined, is the most abundant element next to oxygen in the earth's crust and is used esp. in alloys and electronic devices."

The web site, http://www.anytimevitamins.com/silicon-info.htm, says, "Silicon is used to keep bones, cartilage, tendons and artery walls healthy and may be beneficial in the treatment of allergies, heartburn and gum disease, as well as assisting the immune system." *The site further says,* "It is also required by the nails, hair and skin to stay in good condition and is useful in counteracting the effects of aluminum." [See *"Silicon," in* Chapter 17 titled, *"Conclusion, Putting it all together."*]

Alzheimer's and Aluminum:

Regarding aluminum in the Alzheimer's brain, it is known that when fluoride is added to drinking water, it combines with aluminum to form aluminum fluoride. Hydrochloric stomach acid mixes with the aluminum fluoride, and creates <u>aluminum oxide</u> which can be deposited inside the organs and brain.

Chapter 17 will provide more information on number 14 [Silicon.]

Consider the odds; the odds are astronomical of one element, [number 14, Silicon] out of 114 elements, that can stop the aluminum before it can reach the brain.

Here is the last number.
Number 26 Iron [Fe]

Webster's Dictionary, describes Iron as, "A heavy malleable ductile magnetic silver-white metallic element that readily rusts in moist air, occurs native in meteorites and combined in most igneous rocks, is the most used of metals and is vital to biological processes."

Iron Deficiency and Alzheimer's:

The following article lends support to my research, that, there is an iron [number 26] deficiency in Alzheimer's disease.

An article, by Merritt McKinney, New York Reuters Health, titled, "Iron Deficiency May Contribute To Alzheimer Damage," *reports that,* "New research suggests that a lack of iron may contribute to the decay of brain cells caused by Alzheimer's disease." *The article further says,* "In experiments with human and animal brain cells, reducing the production of the most common form of iron in cells, known as heme, led to degeneration similar to that caused by aging and Alzheimer's disease." *In the article, Dr. Bruce N. Ames, Senior study author, at the Children's Hospital Oakland Research Institute, in California, stated,* "Although, it is too soon to say that getting enough iron will ward off Alzheimer's, there's no excuse for anyone not getting enough iron and other vitamins." *In the interview, Ames said,* "A lack of iron disrupts a person's metabolism by damaging mitochondria, which are the power plants of cells. If mitochondria become damaged, harmful substances called oxidants that can contribute to the aging process can accumulate in cells."

The above article goes on to relate that, *"In experiments directed by first author Hani Atamna, the researchers found that interfering with the production of heme, the form of iron that is essential for normal cell function, caused cells to degenerate and become more likely to die."*

Heme molecule provides Oxygen:

I want to make a point regarding the heme form of iron. This falls under the heading of chelating [a metal ion bonded to at least two non-metal ions.] If we look at the molecular complex of the heme molecule, we find, at the center of the complex an iron atom [atomic number

26.] This iron atom is bonded to nitrogen atoms [atomic number 7.] If one or both of these, iron or nitrogen atoms become <u>inhibited by oxidation</u> caused by methyl-eugenol, and or ethyl-vanillin, the heme molecule could not transport oxygen to the brain. This would result in less cell energy. The Alzheimer's brain is low on cell energy. Hmmm!

Iron and Plaque, are two major players in the Alzheimer's arena:

Iron is important to mental function:

The toxic form of amyloid plaque [A beta 1- 42 peptide,] is found in the Alzheimer's brain and results in cognitive impairment.

Being aware of these two points, consider the statement in the following research dated August 2, 1999, "Alzheimer's Research Forum," by W. Garzon-Rodriguez et. al., Department of Molecular Biology and Biochemistry, University of California at Irvine, USA. States, "The affinity of A beta 1 – 42 for Fe [Iron] increases dramatically upon aggregation." Aha! Think Fenton's Reagent. *[See Chapter 17 titled,* "Conclusion, putting it all together," *and number 26 Iron.]*

Reduced Iron:

The iron is being compromised and not available for mental function. We need iron [number 26] especially for mental health and to carry the oxygen to the brain.

Chapter 17 titled, Conclusion, "Putting It All Together" provides a more scientific explanation of the 6 elements [6 numbers] and exactly how the 6 elements are definitely involved in Alzheimer's dementia.

CHAPTER SIXTEEN:
TO THE POINT

The 7 basic mechanisms
[problems] involved in
Alzheimer's dementia [AD]

Commenting on the testing of non steroidal anti-inflammatory drugs [Nsaids] and published on the Alzforum 25 September 2002, neuroscientist Dr. Monique Breteler related that, "It is highly likely that AB accumulation in the brain does play a central role in Alzheimer's disease. However, what causes this accumulation in the majority of cases is largely unclear. Alzheimer's disease is a multifactorial and heterogeneous disorder. This implies that there is no single cascade of events that ultimately leads to the clinical syndrome. Moreover, it implies that there may be different mechanisms on which one could intervene to prevent or delay onset of disease."

I believe Dr. Breteler's opinion, that there are multiple mechanisms involved in Alzheimer's disease is correct. I will show in this chapter, there are at least 7 mechanisms involved in Alzheimer's disease.

Any therapy that has the ability to reverse Alzheimer's disease must be able to address all seven of these mechanisms. The six mysterious numbers [elements] are involved in all 7 of the following symptoms.

***Stedman's Medical Dictionary describes "mechanism" as,* "the sequence of chemical steps in a chemical reaction."**

The following are the 6 mechanisms [elements] involved in Alzheimer's disease:

[1] Problem: Toxic beta amyloid plaque kills brain cells. There is a lithium deficiency. Lithium #3 is being oxidized. Lithium can block

the GSK-3 protein that aggregates amyloid plaque in the Alzheimer's brain.

[2] Problem: There is a buildup of excess glutamate in the brain cell. There is a nitrogen deficiency. Nitrogen #7 is being oxidized. [The glutamate molecule requires nitrogen.]

[3] Problem: There is a choline deficiency. Choline is needed for the acetylcholine neurotransmitter. There is a nitrogen deficiency. Nitrogen #7 is being oxidized. [The choline molecule requires nitrogen.]

[4] Problem: Oxidative stress causes protein misfolding in the endoplasmic reticulum. There is a fluorine deficiency. Fluorine #9 is being inhibited. [fluorinated alcohol can refold proteins. This requires fluorine.]

[5] Problem: Cell depolarization is inhibited in the Alzheimer's brain resulting in reduced cognition. There is a sodium deficiency. Sodium #11 is being oxidized. [Cell depolarization requires sodium.]

[6] Problem: There is an accumulation of aluminum found in amyloid plaque on postmortem autopsy. There is a silicon deficiency. Silicon #14 is being oxidized. [Aluminum is bound to silicon and then removed from the body. This requires silicon.]

[7] Problem: The Alzheimer's brain is low on cell energy. There is an iron deficiency. Iron #26 is being oxidized. [The heme molecule requires iron to transport oxygen to the mitochondria.]

This neurodegenerative disease terminates with loss of cognition, ending in death and costs society one billion dollars a year.

My findings are, that **[3 - 7 - 9 - 11 - 14 - 26]** represent the atomic elements I need to replace in order to reverse this terrible disease in myself.

Since these numbers [atomic elements] **are definitely involved in Alzheimer's disease,** I believe clinical trials on this will prove me right.

We are faced with two choices here. We can believe I was given these numbers on purpose, to help reverse Alzheimer's dementia or we can believe this occurrence, was a coincidence. If we choose to believe it was coincidental, we must be willing to accept the **astronomical odds of over two and a half billion to one.** [Meaning, choosing the correct six numbers from a total of 114 numbers in the periodic table.] My common sense tells me these odds are next to impossible. It is more logical to believe this information came from a source who knows how to reverse Alzheimer's and who understands what the elements are that are involved in this disease.

I am now 72 years young, I have totally reversed the Alzheimer's dementia in myself and I have continued to stand off this disease for four years now. I know Alzheimer's dementia well. It destroyed my mother's brain, and then started working on mine.

When Alzheimer's dementia started on me, I put everything in my life on hold, including my hobbies, my work, etc. After all, what is there to life if a person loses their memory? Stopping this disease became the number one priority in my life. Therefore, I sat down and started reading, day and night, seven days a week. Seven years later, I have over 90 % of this disease figured out.

I want to share this information with you. I read food labels, if it contains eugenol, methyl-eugenol, ethyl-vanillin, vanillin [artificial flavors], vanilla extract and double emulsifiers, I try not to put it into my body. I hate to tell you this, but, this eliminates a large part of the foods on the grocery store shelves. We can't go wrong eating fresh fruits and vegetables.

Artificial flavors are cheaper to produce compared to natural flavors.

On the other hand, I have eaten these products most all my life with no memory problems what so ever. However, things changed when I reached 65 years of age. Now ethyl-vanillin [a triple strength oxidizer] combined with double strength emulsifiers [two emulsifiers] and vanilla extract, can overpower my age weakened biochemical system.

Eugenol is used in dentistry and is an oxidizer. Clove oil is 85% eugenol. Remember the old Red Cross toothache medicine that blocked nerve transmission of pain? Well, it contains 85% Eugenol. Hmm! Blocks the nerve transmission of pain! Nerve transmission is also blocked in Alzheimer's disease.

Think about it! Vanillin is distilled from methyl-eugenol and it is an oxidizer.

Where would you find most of these artificial flavors, ethyl vanillin, vanilla extract and emulsifiers? They are found in desserts, cookies, and candy and bakery products like donuts, cakes, pies and especially in ice cream, milk shakes and malts.

Numerous studies report that, people who consume the most calories are at the greatest risk of developing Alzheimer's disease. But, my findings are, it's not the calories that caused my memory deficit, it just happens that the foods which contain the most calories also contain methyl-eugenol, ethyl-vanillin and vanillin [artificial flavors] vanilla extract and emulsifiers.

Think about it! Fat kids do not get Alzheimer's disease, because their biochemical systems have not started to weaken from old age.

After years of trying to put all of this together, I finally figured out all I had to do to reverse this memory deficit in myself was to remove the methyl-eugenol, ethyl-vanillin [artificial flavors,] vanilla extract and double emulsifiers from my diet. I also replaced artificially flavored drinks with naturally flavored drinks. Fresh fruit, vegetables and nuts [Mediterranean diet] are free of these chemical additives. That is one reason they are good for us older folks.

I take the anti-oxidant vitamins A, C, and E plus a good multiple B vitamin complex.

Most important of all, I take two or three _trace mineral supplements_ a day that contain the elements: lithium, nitrogen, fluoride/fluorine, sodium, silicon, and iron. The reason these *"six trace elements"* must be replaced, is because, the artificial flavors, [methyl-eugenol, ethyl-vanillin,] combined with vanilla extract and emulsifiers are oxidizing these very important trace mineral elements in my body.

Studies show a 79% reduction in the onset of Alzheimer's disease in people taking Statins.

Ask your doctor about Statins. Lipitor is one example. Lipitor contains fluorine, [number 9], which is not available over the counter. [Fluoride is the reduced form of fluorine, and is available over the counter in supplement form.] Lipitor also contains the element nitrogen [number 7], another element that I need to replace on a continual basis for a good memory.

Studies also show that oxidative stress is a major problem for Alzheimer's patients, because it causes protein misfolding. Guess what? Ethyl vanillin is a triple strength oxidizer. Think about it!

Better yet, do what I did. Go to your local bakery and ask to see the gallon container they use for artificial vanilla flavoring in almost all their donuts, rolls, etc. The label will say propylene-glycol, ethyl-vanillin. **Propylene-glycol is an emulsifier-solvent and ethyl-vanillin is a triple strength oxidizer.** Vanilla extract is also used.

I don't think these are a problem for younger people, because they never caused me problems when I was younger, as far as I know.

Why is the triple strength oxidizer a problem for my memory? Because, it is oxidizing very important *"trace mineral elements"* needed for my normal cognition. This oxidation also creates free radicals. Vitamins, A, C, and E are needed as antioxidants to counteract the free radicals.

When I replace the *"six elements,"* on a regular basis, my memory remains as good as ever.

Studies show that adding fresh fruits, vegetables and nuts to our diet is beneficial in warding off Alzheimer's disease. Why is this beneficial? Because, fruits, vegetables and nuts contain the *"six elements"* lithium, nitrogen, fluorine/fluoride, sodium, silicon and iron which need to be replaced so my brain can function properly.

Simply put, I try to stay away from all forms of eugenol, ethyl-vanillin [artificial flavors], combined with double emulsifiers and vanilla extract.

Think Trace Mineral Replacement:

I take Trace Mineral Supplements which contain the *"six atomic elements"* [numbers] that are listed in *"The Periodic Table of Elements,"* as follows:

Number   3 [Lithium.]
Number   7 [Nitrogen.]
Number   9 [Fluorine/Fluoride.]
Number 11 [Sodium.]
Number 14 [Silicon.]
Number 26 [Iron.]

To learn more, see our web site at, **www.zapalzheimers.com**

Number 9 [Fluorine], is not available over the counter, but the reduced form, fluoride is. Fluorine is available in Lipitor and some other statins. Again, talk to your doctor regarding this.

I take a good multiple Vitamin-B complex that contain:

B- 1 [Thiamin.]
B- 2 [Riboflavin.]
B- 3 [Niacin.]
B- 5 [Pantothenic acid.]
B- 6 [Pyridoxine.]
B- 9 [Folic acid.]
B-12 [Cobalamin.]

This is all I have to do to reverse the memory deficit in myself. If I do not do these things, then Alzheimer's starts coming back and my memory and cognition starts to decline. This was the way Alzheimer's disease gradually destroyed Mother's brain, over a nine or ten year period. Depriving her of the ability to pray for guidance and forgiveness. Not to mention, being unable to enjoy the twilight years of her life.

Let's look at this using two of the greatest assets we have, human intuition and good old fashioned common sense.

Alzheimer's disease is worldwide, so whatever the cause, it must also be worldwide. Methyl-eugenol and propylene-glycol, ethyl-vanillin production fits this requirement because they are also produced worldwide along with the emulsifiers.

Next, look at the studies on alcohol and Alzheimer's disease. Studies show that one or two drinks a day fend off Alzheimer's disease. Methyl-eugenol and ethyl-vanillin are practicably non-water soluble. However, they are soluble in alcohol. This tells me a couple of drinks a day reduce Alzheimer's symptoms by diluting the methyl-eugenol and ethyl-vanillin.

Look at the studies on calories. Studies show the less calories a person consumes, the less they are at risk of Alzheimer's disease. If we look at the foods which contain the most calories, we find they are desserts. These desserts contain methyl-eugenol, ethyl-vanillin, double emulsifiers and vanilla extract. It's not the calories that are the problem. They just happen to be in the same areas of food that contains the methyl-eugenol, ethyl-vanillin, double emulsifiers and vanilla extract.

Let's look at oxidative stress that causes protein misfolding in multiple neurodegenerative diseases like the Alzheimer's disease. Methyl-eugenol and ethyl-vanillin are known oxidizers. It clearly says so on their packaging labels. "Keep away from light, air and do not put in steel or metal containers." Why? Because, to expose these chemicals to light and oxygen will cause metals to oxidize and this will eat holes in the metal containers.

Oxidized copper, zinc and manganese.

How about oxidized iron, also?

Two of the major problems in neurodegenerative diseases, are sod mutants that lose their ability to scavenge free radicals and, a lack of oxygen to the mitochondria, which results in less adenosine triphosphate [ATP] being produced.

See how <u>methyl-eugenol and ethyl-vanillin are</u> <u>responsible for</u> <u>oxidizing metals?</u> This oxidation also results in oxidative stress in the endoplasmic reticulum that is causing protein misfolding.

Think about this. <u>Oxidation, caused by methyl-eugenol, ethyl-</u><u>vanillin, oxidizes copper, zinc and manganese and releases free radicals</u><u>that interfere with the free radical control of the super oxide dismutase</u><u>[SOD] protein,</u> both in the cell nucleus and the cytoplasm of the cell.

Dr. Elmer M. Cranton, states in his fine book titled, **"Bypassing Bypass** **Surgery,"** *that,* "Concentration of the free radical control enzyme, superoxide dismutase [SOD] in mammels is directly proportional to life span."

Dr. Cranton also says in his book that, "Copper, zinc and manganese are all essential for super oxide dismutase activity. Free radical damage in the brain and central nervous system [CNS] can be assessed by the rate of cholesterol depletion."

Propylene glycol is both an emulsifier and a solvent. An emulsifier allows water and oils [fats] to mix. Vitamins are needed for the proper function of enzymes. Vitamins are either water-soluble or fat-soluble.

My common sense tells me that a double strength emulsifier that allows water and oils to mix, may be interfering with the proper use of vitamins, sending water soluble vitamins and fat soluble vitamins to areas not intended. This could interfere with an enzymes ability to rapidly catalyze biochemical reactions in a weakened biochemical system of an elderly person.

So, after years of research and testing on myself, here is my view of the pathogenesis of my Alzheimer's disease.

As time goes by and my body ages, certain atomic elements are inhibited by the combined process of **oxidation and emulsification.** There is a small deficiency of a select group of vitamins, trace elements and certain minerals, allowing memory problems to appear.

Mild cognitive impairment [MCI] is the diagnosis.

The amount of the element and vitamin deficiency depends upon the consumption of artificial flavors combined with emulsifiers. The older the body, the weaker will become the biochemical defense and immune system. As more time goes by, vitamins, trace elements and certain minerals continue to be depleted even more. Memory problems increase. The disease advances.

Moderate Alzheimer's disease is now the diagnosis.

As years go by, my body grows older and its biochemical system weakens even more. Additional, artificial flavors combined with emulsifiers are now able to inhibit even more of these very necessary vitamins, trace elements and certain minerals. When the necessary amount of vitamins, trace elements and certain minerals are unavailable to act as co-factors for the enzymes that catalyze biochemical reactions, we now enter advanced cognitive impairment.

If these very important vitamins, trace elements and certain minerals are not replaced, they will become even more depleted.

Severe Alzheimer's disease is now the diagnosis.

Unless, this deficiency is corrected by replacing the inhibited vitamins and certain atomic elements, along with removing these oxidizers and emulsifiers from the diet, this condition will eventually end in death just like Mothers, did. **Severe Alzheimer's disease.**

I know that for the lay person [like me] some of this book is hard to understand. That is why I wrote this Chapter titled, *"To The Point"* for you. If you will study these few pages, you may find the information you are searching for.

For more information visit our web site at www.zapalzheimers.com.

Give thanks to our Creator for he truly is
The Master Intelligence of the Universe that
"Causes to be."

CHAPTER SEVENTEEN: CONCLUSION, PUTTING IT ALL TOGETHER

In this chapter, I will use science to detail the numbers and how they are involved in Alzheimer's disease. **These numbers represent** *"Six elements"* **in the** *"Periodic Table of Elements."*

Neuroscientists all over the world are working to find the correct therapy that will reverse Alzheimer's disease.

I want to share my work in the hope that together, we can bring this terrible disease under control or end it completely.

My research reveals Alzheimer's to be a disease of element deficiency. Certain elements in my aged body are being oxidized. This produces free radicals and ionic inhibition of the "six very important atomic elements." *Vitamins, are also being inhibited.*

THE OXIDATION OF METALS AND THE
EMULSIFICATION OF VITAMINS

After 7 years of Alzheimer's research, my findings are that **dementia and cognitive impairment appear** when the age weakened biochemical system in the body can no longer handle **two combined chemicals in food and drink.** These two chemicals are **artificial flavors,** which are **oxidizers,** combined with **emulsifiers,** which **allow water and oils to mix.**

These **oxidizers** are eugenol, methyl eugenol, iso eugenol, ethyl vanillin and vanillin. They are listed on food labels as **artificial flavors.** They will accumulate in an elderly person's body **and oxidize the metals** contained in the metalloproteins, kicking off free radicals which are unpaired electrons. This, process inhibits the enzymes ability to catalyze biochemical reactions.

<u>Artificial flavors also oxidize</u> the atomic elements of lithium, nitrogen, fluorine, sodium, silicon and iron. Oxidation of copper, zinc and manganese inhibits the function of the free radical scavenger "super oxide dismutase" [SOD], thereby rendering it ineffective.

<u>Emulsifiers</u> such as propylene glycol and soya lecithin allow fats [oils] and water to mix. Vitamins are either water soluble or fat soluble. Vitamins act as cofactors for enzymes, allowing them to rapidly synthesize biochemical reactions, unless they are confused by multiple emulsifiers. Propylene glycol-ethyl vanillin is an emulsifier solvent and a double strength oxidizer. They are found in candy, ice cream, bakery products, desserts and soft drinks.

The following are some of the problems caused by the combining of artificial flavors with emulsifiers in elderly people's diet: Amyloid plaque forms in the brain; <u>Calcium</u> and <u>glutamate</u> build up in the cell; the amino acid <u>tryptophan</u> is mutated, inhibiting <u>serotonin, niacin</u> and <u>melatonin;</u> the <u>choline molecule</u> is mutated, causing a choline deficiency which inhibits the <u>acetylcholine neurotransmitter.</u>

Consider all the advice we receive regarding oxidation and antioxidants.

Webster's Dictionary describes antioxidant as, "A substance that inhibits oxidation or reactions promoted by oxygen or peroxides." Neuroscientists worldwide are also studying oxidative stress and its effect on the Alzheimer's brain and other neurodegenerative diseases.

Unless otherwise noted, additional information on the following published neuroscience research papers can be found online at, the *Alzheimer's Research Forum.* This is a centralized location for the publication of research papers dealing with Alzheimer's and other neurodegenerative diseases.

So what do Neuroscientists worldwide say about Oxidation?

Oxidation, Lipids and Lipoproteins:

2001, August

Dr. A. Kontush et al of the Clinic of Internal Medicine, University Hospital, Hamburg, Germany, reports in their research that, "Increased oxidation is an important feature of Alzheimer's disease [AD] and major targets for oxidation in the brain are lipids and lipoproteins."

Oxidation and Aging:
2001, December

Dr. S. Arlt et. al., and Associates of the Institut fur Medizinische Biochemie und Molekularbiologie Hamburg, Germany, reports in their research that, "Oxidative processes are involved in aging as well as the pathogenesis of different degenerative diseases."

Oxidative damage in the Alzheimer's brain:
2002, May

Dr. M. Grundman et. al., of the Alzheimer's disease Cooperative Study, University of California, San Diego, USA, reports that, "Oxidative damage is present within the brains of patients with Alzheimer's disease [AD], and is observed within every class of biomolecule."

Oxidative Stress:
2004, March

Dr. C. Moreno-Sanchez et.al., of the Nutrition and Neurocognition Laboratory on Aging Research Center, Tufts University, Boston, Ma, USA, reports in their research that, "Oxidative stress is an important trigger in the complex chain of events leading to neurodegenerative diseases."

Free radical lipid peroxidation:
2004

Dr. A. Tappel, of the Department of Food Science and Technology, University of California, Davis, Ca. USA, reports in research titled, "Oxidant free radical initiated chain polymerization of protein and other biomolecules and its relationship to disease," Dr. Tappel says, "Free radical lipid peroxidation could initiate the chain polymerization of amyloid peptides and other biomolecules found in Alzheimer's disease."

So, regarding Alzheimer's, what are the elements being oxidized and what are the processes by which this occurs? First, let us look at the elements that are being oxidized.

They are **3 – 7 – 9 – 11 – 14 – 26.** "The numbers represent atomic elements in *"The Periodic Table of Elements,"* that I need to replace on a continual basis in order to maintain a good memory.

The first number.
Number 3 represents Lithium [Li]

Stedman's Medical Dictionary describes Lithium as "A soft highly reactive metallic element. Atomic number 3." Oxidize lithium and we get lithium oxide. Lithium is then inhibited and needs to be replaced.

So what do neuroscientists say about Alzheimer's disease and replacing lithium?

Lithium, a selective inhibitor of GSK-3 beta:
2001, November

Dr. C.A. Grimes and Dr. R.S. Jope of the Department of Psychiatry and Behavioral Neurobiology, University of Alabama at Birmingham AL. USA. reports that, "Glycogen synthase kinase-3beta [GSK-3beta] is a fascinating enzyme with an astoundingly diverse number of actions in intracellular signaling systems. Lithium, the primary therapeutic agent for bipolar mood disorder, is a selective inhibitor of GSK-3beta." *Grimes and Jope also reported that,* "GSK-3beta has been linked to all of the primary abnormalities associated with Alzheimer's disease."

Lithium inhibits increase in tau phosphorylation:
2002, May

Dr. W. Elyaman and Associates of the Department of Anatomy, Faculty of Medicine, The University of Hong Kong, Hong Kong, SAR reports that, "The dissociation of the neuronal Golgi complex is a classical feature observed in neurodegenerative disorders including Alzheimer's disease." *Reporting further on their test results, the team relates that,* "The increase in tau phosphorylation was inhibited by the GSK-3 inhibitor, lithium. Finally, morphometric studies showed that lithium partially blocked the Golgi disassembly."

Accumulation of the beta-amyloid characterizes Alzheimer's:
2002, June

Dr. G. Alvarez and Associates of Departmento de Biologia Molecular, Centro de Biologia Molecular Severo Ochoa Universidad Autonoma de Madrid, Madrid, Spain, reports that, "Alzheimer's disease is a neurodegenerative disorder characterized by the accumulation of the beta-amyloid peptide and the hyperphosphorylation of the tau protein, among other features." *They further report that,* "In our opinion the possibility of using lithium, or other inhibitors of glycogen synthase kinase-3, in experimental trials aimed to ameliorate neurodegeneration in Alzheimer's disease should be considered."

Lithium blocks accumulation of abeta peptides:
2003, May

Dr. C.J. Phiel and Associates, of Dr. P.S. Klein, of the Department of Medicine, Division of Hematology-Oncology and Howard Hughes Medical Institute, University of Pennsylvania School of Medicine, Philadelphia, Penn. USA, reports that, "Alzheimer's disease is associated with increased production and aggregation of amyloid beta [Abeta] peptides." *The team further reports that,* "Importantly, lithium also blocks the accumulation of Abeta peptides in the brains of mice that overproduce APP." *[Author-APP is the abbreviation for amyloid precursor protein.]*

Lithium reduces abeta production:
2003, December

Dr. J. Ryder and Associates of Neuroscience Discovery Research, Lilly Research Laboratories, Indianapolis, Indiana, USA, reports that, "Oral administration of lithium significantly reduces Abeta production." [Authors note: Abeta production is the aggregation of Beta Amyloid plaque that forms in the Alzheimer's brain.]

Lithium reduces neuron damage:
2004, April

Dr. V. V. Senatorov et. al., of the Molecular Neurobiology section, National Institute of Mental Health, Bethesda, MD, USA. reports, "Lithium significantly diminished the loss of neurons in animal testing and lithium also reduced the number of neurons showing DNA damage or activated caspase-3." *[Authors note: caspase-3 involves apoptosis or programmed cell death.]*

The total focus seems to be on adding lithium to the diet. Obviously, one must ask, what is wrong with the lithium already in our diet, and why does it need to be replaced?

Think oxidation.

The second number.
Number 7 represents Nitrogen [N]

Stedman's Medical Dictionary, describes Nitrogen as, "A nonmetallic element that constitutes nearly four fifths of the air by volume, occurring as a colorless, odorless, almost inert diatomic gas N2, in various minerals and in all proteins. Atomic number 7."

Oxidation and negative nitrogen balance:

Oxidize nitrogen and we get nitric oxide. Nitrogen is then inhibited and needs to be replaced. If nitrogen needs to be replaced, would not this condition create, "Negative nitrogen balance?"

Mosby's Medical Dictionary, Sixth Edition states, "Negative nitrogen balance occurs when more nitrogen is excreted then is taken in, and indicates wasting or destruction of tissue."

Whether nitrogen is excreted or inhibited, a deficiency exists. When you consider that nitrogen plays a major role in proteins and amino acid synthesis, destruction of tissue results in inflammation and what treats inflammation? Non-steroidal anti-inflammatory drugs, [Nsaids!] It all fits!

According to Webster's Dictionary, "Nitric oxide is a colorless poisonous gas NO formed by oxidation of nitrogen or ammonia."

**So what do neuroscientists say about nitrogen,
oxidation and Alzheimer's disease?**

Reactive nitrogen species:

2001, December

Dr. J. P. Blass, of the Weill Cornell Medical College, at the Burke Medical Research Institute, White Plains, NY, reports that, "The potential of impairments in oxidative/energy metabolism to cause diseases of the brain had been proposed even before the major pathways of oxidative/

energy metabolism were described. Deficiencies associated with disease are known in all the pathways of oxidative/energy metabolism and are associated with some of the most common disorders of the nervous system, including Alzheimer's disease [AD] and Parkinson's disease [PD.]" *Dr. Blass also reports that,* "A common mechanism in these conditions appears to be a downward mitochondrial spiral, involving abnormalities in energy metabolism, calcium metabolism, and free radicals."

A downward mitochondrial spiral, involving abnormalities in energy metabolism, calcium metabolism, and free radicals?

Energy metabolism in the mitochondria involves the heme molecule because; it carries oxygen to the mitochondria. If we look at the molecular complex of the heme molecule what we find is a central iron atom [atomic number 26] bonded to four nitrogen atoms [atomic number 7.] Now stop and think about this. When one understands that methyl-eugenol and ethyl-vanillin are major oxidizers the picture becomes clearer. Oxidize the iron atom and or the nitrogen atom in the heme molecule and the transportation of oxygen to the mitochondria is inhibited. This results in abnormalities in energy metabolism. It also explains the source of the free radicals.

Thinking about the inhibition of the iron and or the nitrogen atom in the heme molecular complex, *Cliffs AP Biology, Second Edition, page 75, says,* "If no oxygen is delivered to the mitochondria, the Krebs cycle and glycolysis both stop and the cell dies." Cells in the Alzheimer's brain also die. It all fits, doesn't it?

Calcium is listed as a metal in the "Periodic Table of Elements." Metals can be oxidized presenting more free radicals to deal with. We can tie this in with the non evasive scan for calcium used to locate blocked arteries. See how oxidation, Alzheimer's and heart disease are linked together.

What comes to mind is that calcium signals through the transduction pathway, unless of course it is inhibited by oxidation.

Alzheimer's disease involves neuronal cell dysfunction:
2002, March-April

Dr. C. Behl and Dr. B. Moosmann, of the Max-Planck-Institute of Psychiatry, Munich, Germany, reports that,

"Many neurodegenerative disorders and syndromes are associated with an excessive generation of reactive oxygen species [ROS] and oxidative stress." *They further report that,* "In Alzheimer's disease [AD] oxidative neuronal cell dysfunction and cell death caused by protofibrils and aggregates of the AD-associated amyloid beta protein [Abeta] may causally contribute to pathogenesis and progression. ROS and reactive nitrogen species also take part in the complex cascade of events and the detrimental effects occurring during ischemia and reperfusion in stroke."

Reactive nitrogen oxide species:

2002, may

Dr. M. G. Espey and Associates, of the Radiation Biology Branch, National Cancer Institute, National Institutes of Health, Bethesda, Maryland, report that, "Nitric oxide [nitrogen monoxide NO] plays a veritable cornucopia of regulatory roles in normal physiology. In contrast, NO has also been implicated in the etiology and sequela of numerous neurodegenerative diseases that involve reactive oxygen species [ROS] and reactive nitrogen oxide species [RNOS.]" *Author: See how oxidized nitrogen impacts neurodegenerative diseases.*

Oxidation by reactive nitrogen species:

2003, April

Dr. M.Z. Wrona et. al., of the Department of Chemistry and Biochemistry, University of Oklahoma, Norman, Oklahoma, reports that, "Tryptamine-4-5-dione [1] is formed by oxidation of the neurotransmitter 5-hydroxytryptamine by reactive oxygen and reactive nitrogen species and on the basis of in vitro and in vivo studies, it has been proposed to be a neurotoxin that may contribute to the selective neurodegeneration in Alzheimer's disease and serotonergic neurotoxicity of methamphetamine."

Author: See how the essential amino acid tryptophan is mutated. This inhibits the function of the neurotransmitter serotonin, and also niacin, and melatonin.

Cross talk between copper, zinc and the SOD mutant:

2003 June

Dr. K. Aquilano and Associates at the Department of Biology, University of Rome Tor Vergata, Rome, Italy, reports that, "Reactive oxygen and nitrogen species have emerged as predominant effectors of neurodegeneration." *They report further that,* "Overall their tests results confirm the pro-oxidant activity of G93A Cu, Zn, SOD mutant and, at the same time, suggest cross talk between reactive oxygen and nitrogen species."

Author: A sod mutant is also involved in other neurodegenerative diseases, say like Amyotrophic Lateral Sclerosis [ALS.]

Reactive nitrogen species inhibits fibril formation:

2003, June

Dr. H. Ischiropoulos, of the Stokes Research Institute, Department of Biochemistry and Biophysics, Children's Hospital of Philadelphia and University of Pennsylvania, Philadelphia, Pennsylvania, reports that, "Hallmark lesions of neurodegenerative synucleinopathies contain alpha-synuclein [alpha-syn] that is modified by nitration of tyrosine residues and possibly by dityrosine cross linking to generated stable oligomers." *Dr. Ischiropoulos further relates that,* "Posttranslational modifications of alpha-syn by reactive nitrogen species inhibit fibril formation and results in urea-and SDS-insoluble, protease-

resistant alpha-syn aggregates that may be responsible for cellular toxicity."

A problem with tyrosine, is a problem for dopamine, is a problem for Parkinsons disease.

Reactive nitrogen oxide species. Neuroprotection or neurotoxicity:

2004, January

Dr. K.M. Boje of the Department of Pharmaceutical Sciences, School of Pharmacy and Pharmaceutical Sciences, University at Buffalo, Buffalo, NY. reports that, "Nitric oxide [Nitrogen monoxide; NO] is a simple molecule with diverse biological functions. NO and related reactive nitrogen oxide species [RNOS] mediate intricate physiological and pathophysiological effects in the central nervous system. Depending on environmental conditions, NO and RNOS can initiate and mediate neuroprotection or neurotoxicity either exclusively or synergistically with other effectors."

Is oxidized nitrogen a problem for elderly people? I think so.

Reactive nitrogen species, oxidative stress, and protein misfolding:

2004, January

Dr. J. Emerit et, al., of the Service des Maladies Infectieuses et Tropicales, Groupe Hospitalier Pitie-Salpetriere 47, boulevard de l'Hospital, Paris, France, reports that, "Oxidative stress is now recognized as accountable for redox regulation involving reactive oxygen species [ROS] and reactive nitrogen species [RNS.] Its role is pivotal for the modulation of critical cellular functions, notably for neurons astrocytes and microglia, such as apoptosis program activation, and ion transport, calcium mobilization, involved in excitotoxicity." *Dr. Emerit and the team further relate that,* "The cascade of events that leads to neurons death is complex. In addition to mitochondrial dysfunction [apoptosis,] excitotoxicity, oxidative stress [inflammation,] the mechanisms from gene to disease involve also protein misfolding leading to aggregates and proteasome dysfunction on ubiquinited material."

Reactive nitrogen species involved in neurodegeneration:

2004, May-June

Dr. V. Calabrese and Associates, of the Section of Biochemistry and Molecular Biology, Department of Chemistry, Faculty of Medicine, University of Catania, Catania, Italy, report that, "Nitric oxide and other reactive nitrogen species appear to play crucial roles in the brain such as neuromodulation, neurotransmission and synaptic plasticity, but are also involved in pathological processes such as neurodegeneration and neuroinflammation. Acute and chronic inflammation results in increased nitrogen monoxide formation and nitrosative stress." *Dr. Calabrese and the team further relate that,* "It is now well documented that NO and its toxic metabolite, peroxynitrite, can inhibit components of the mitochondrial respiratory chain leading to cellular energy deficiency and eventually, to cell death."

Author: So we see that nitric oxide reduces cell energy and triggers cell death.

So if molecules containing oxidized nitrogen are inhibited, then the nitrogen [atomic number 7] must be replaced.

The third number.
Number 9 represents Fluorine [F]

Stedman's Medical Dictionary, describes Fluorine *as,* "A highly corrosive poisonous gaseous halogen element, the most reactive of all the elements."

Studies show that cholesterol lowering statins offer a 79% reduction in the onset of Alzheimer's disease. **The statins, Crestor, Lipitor, and Vytorin contain the element fluorine, [*Atomic number 9.*]**

Nitrogen, [atomic number 7] is also contained in these statin drugs. Is this why they are partially effective against Alzheimer's disease?

Isn't the reason these 3 statin drugs reduce the chances of getting Alzheimer's disease, is because, fluorine is refolding proteins and nitrogen is removing the mutation from the choline molecule enabling acetylcholine neurotransmitter function, not to mention that replacing the nitrogen in amino acids improves bio synthesis.

Fluorine is still somewhat of a puzzle to me in that I have not been able to find much published research regarding fluorine and Alzheimer's disease. One thing I am sure of though, I would bet the farm, that fluorine/fluoride needs to be replaced because replacing all of the *"six elements"* completely reversed all my Alzheimer's symptoms.

Fluoride, the reduced form of fluorine is available over the counter in supplement form.

Alzheimer's disease and
Over-firing of neurons linked to cell death:
1999

Dr. Adeboye Adejare of the Department of Pharmaceutical Sciences, College of Pharmacy, Pocatello, Idaho, USA, reports that, "Their earlier work focussed on adrenergic receptors, including how location of fluorine on adrenergic ligands can be used to obtain selectivity between the various receptors." *Adejare relates that,* "Over firing of neurons has been linked to neuronal degeneration and cell death as observed in stroke and Alzheimer's disease."

Protein misfolding:

Regarding fluorine, consider the above research [in nitrogen number 7] *2004 January, of Dr. J. Emerit and the team as they related that,* "The mechanisms from gene to disease involve also protein misfolding."

Consider the following research that also deals with protein misfolding.

Fluorinated alcohols can refold the beta-conformation:

2003, January

Dr. E. P. Vieira, Dr. H. Hermel and Dr. H. Mohwald of the Max-Planck-Institute for Colloids and Interfaces, Campus Golm, Potsdam, Germany, reports that, "Change and stabilization of the amyloid-beta [1-40] secondary structure by fluorocompounds." *The team further relates that,* "The misfolding of the amyloid peptide, which is the result of a well-known alpha-to-beta transition, causes neurodegenerative disorder." *Vieira and the team further relate that,* "Fluorinated alcohols have been described in the literature as potent solvents which can refold the beta-conformation. The present studies demonstrate the effectiveness of differently fluorinated alcohols for the beta-to-alpha refolding process on fibrillar aggregated amyloid beta [1-40.]" *The team concludes that,* "Therefore, the use of fluorine groups in the development of new drugs is considered a new possibility requiring further investigation for the prevention of amyloidosis."

Use of fluorine groups and new drugs?
Misfolded proteins lead to cellular damage and death:

2004, September 10,

Dr. C. M. Haynes et. al., of the Division of Cell Biology and Biophysics, School of Biological Sciences, University of Missouri-Kansas City, Kansas, USA relates that, "A variety of debilitating diseases including Diabetes, Alzheimer's, Huntington's, Parkinson's, and prion-based disease are linked to stress within the endoplasmic reticulum [ER.]" *Haynes and the team conclude,* "Our results demonstrate a direct mechanism [s] by which misfolded proteins lead to cellular damage and death."

The point is, fluorinated alcohols can refold proteins. Would not fluorine be needed to synthesize fluorinated alcohols?

Fluorine is the most electronegative of the 114 known elements. This electronegativity is needed to properly synthesize biochemical reactions. [Attract electrons.]

Fluorine is also used in the synthesis of Fluoxetine [Prozac.] *Webster's Dictionary describes Fluoxetine as,* "An anti-depressant drug that enhances serotonin activity." Remember that, serotonin is inhibited because of the mutated amino acid tryptophan. See how important fluorine/fluoride is in biochemical synthesis, concerning Alzheimer's disease.

What is wrong with the fluorine we have from our diet? Why does it have to be replaced? **Think propylene-glycol, ethyl-vanillin. [emulsifier, solvent, and oxidizers]**

The fourth number.
Number 11 represents Sodium [Na]

Stedman's Medical Dictionary describes Sodium as, "A soft, light, highly reactive metallic element that is naturally abundant, especially in common salt. Atomic number 11."

Our brain cells would not function without sodium:

2004 May

Titled, "Brevetoxin activation of voltage-gated sodium channels regulates Ca dynamics and ERK1/2 phosphorylation in murine neocortical neurons." S.M. Dravid et. al., *of the University of Georgia, says,* "Voltage-gated sodium channels [VGSC] are involved in the generation of action potentials in neurons."

Stedman's Medical Dictionary describes Action Potential as, "The change in membrane potential occurring in nerve, muscle or other excitable tissue when excitation occurs."

Several over the counter anti-inflammatory drugs contain sodium. One example is Aleve. It contains 220 mg of naproxen sodium. Sodium is number 11 in *"The Periodic Table of Elements."* According to

Dr.Koop.com, "The body uses sodium to regulate blood pressure and blood volume. Sodium is also critical for the functioning of muscles and nerves."

Sodium ions are vital:

The Chlorine Chemistry Council says, "Our body's cells exist in a sea of fluid. This extracellular body fluid is mostly water, along with the charged atoms [ions] of sodium and chloride. Chloride and other chlorine compounds play an essential role in a delicate balancing act: providing for the electrical neutrality and the correct pressure for the body fluids, and in keeping the acid-base balance of the body." *The Council further relates that,* "Sodium ions are vital to the transmission of impulses from the brain to our muscles through the complex network of nerve cells."

Sodium is used by the the sodium potassium pump that moves ions in and out of our nerve cells.

So the bottom line here is, sodium is a metal, and metals can be oxidized. Oxidation creates free radicals [the reason we need the anti-oxidant vitamins, A, C, and E] and inhibits the function of sodium by interfering with neuron transmission. [Synaptic currents.]

If sodium [number 11] is inhibited, then it needs to be replaced:

The fifth number.
Number 14 represents Silicon [Si]

Stedman's Medical Dictionary, says, "Silicon is a nonmetallic element occurring extensively in the earth's crust in silica and silicates, having both an amorphous and a crystalline allotrope and used in glass and semi conducting devices. Atomic number 14."

Aluminum is found in high concentrations in the Alzheimer's brain. The following report confirms this. Whether it directly contributes to Alzheimer's disease is still being debated. One thing is clear though, it should not be there.

High concentrations of aluminum found in plaques:
1986

Titled, "*Aluminosilicates and the ageing brain: implications for the pathogenesis of Alzheimer's disease.*" *Dr.J. A. Edwardson and Associates states,* "Senile plaques are a neuropathological feature of the ageing brain and consist of abnormal neuritic and glial processes surrounding an extracellular core of material with fibrillary ultra structure." *The team further relates that,* "Isolated cores and plaques in situ from patients with Alzheimer's disease or Down's syndrome and from normal controls have shown co-localization of high concentrations of aluminum [4-19%] and silicon [6-24%] at the centre of the core."

In my opinion from the above information, it appears that silicon was trying to attach to the aluminum in order to remove it, and was caught up in the sticky beta amyloid plaque. The following report shows the affinity silicon [number 14] has for aluminum, or is at the very least trying to remove it from the body.

Silicon reduces gastrointestinal aluminum absorption:
1998

Titled "Silicon reduces aluminum accumulation in rats: relevance to the aluminum hypothesis of Alzheimer disease." Doctor M. Belles et. al., of the School of Medicine, Rovira I Virgili University, Reus, Spain, relates that, "In recent years, a possible relation between the aluminum and silicon levels in drinking water and the risk of Alzheimer's disease [AD] has been established. It has been suggested that silicon may have a protective effect in limiting oral aluminum absorption." *The team further relates that,* "The present study was undertaken to examine the influence of supplementing silicon in the diet to prevent tissue aluminum retention in rats exposed to oral aluminum." *Reporting further on their test results the team states,* "The current results corroborate that silicon effectively prevents gastrointestinal aluminum absorption, which may be of concern in protecting against the neurotoxic effects of aluminum."

I want to repeat the above research,

"The current results corroborate that <u>Silicon effectively prevents</u> gastrointestinal <u>Aluminum absorption.</u>"

The following report speaks of silicon and lithium. **Silicon and lithium are protective.**

Ultra *"trace elements"* are currently being studied:

2002

Titled, "Silicon, aluminum, arsenic and lithium: essentiality and human health implications."

Dr. Granados-Perez and Associates, of the Institute of Nutrition Ciudad Universitaria, Madrid, Spain reports that, "Ultratrace elements are currently being studied to determine their nutritional significance and impact on health, taking into account their possible toxic effects. Some elements are essential to one or more specific biological functions in humans while other is nonessential." *In summation, the team relates that* "Silicon and lithium are protective while aluminum and arsenic have toxic effects."

Oxidized lithium and silicon:

Lithium in the *"Periodic Table of Elements"* is

[Atomic number 3,] Here again lithium is a metal. If it is oxidized, its function is inhibited and it needs to be replaced. Research shows that replacing lithium blocks the GSK-3 protein thereby blocking the aggregation of the amyloid plaque. Common sense alone dictates that if we have lithium and silicon along with the other four elements in our bodies, why do they have to be replaced? The only logical answer is, they are being oxidized and/or inhibited by artificial flavors, emulsifiers and solvents in our food supply which is causing dementia in older people whose biochemical system has weakened from aging.

Aluminum oxide:

A test I have conducted regarding oxidized aluminum, reveals that aluminum can be leached out from aluminum foil by exposing it to propylene-glycol [emulsifier and solvent] and ethyl-vanillin [triple strength oxidizer] and light [electromagnetic radiation.]

You can view a photograph of the test results on our web site located at www.zapalzheimers.com

What about aluminum baking pans? I believe this is another way aluminum is finding its way into the gastrointestinal tract.

The above research shows replacing silicon [atomic number 14] blocks the gastrointestinal absorption of the aluminum, and removes the aluminum from the body before it can reach the brain.

The sixth number.
Number 26 represents Iron [Fe]

Stedman's Medical Dictionary describes Iron as "A lustrous, malleable, ductile, magnetic or magnetizable metallic element. Atomic number 26." *It further says,* "A pill or other medication containing iron and taken as a dietary supplement."

How important is iron to the brain? The following neuroscience research reports answers this question.

Ferritin synthesis severely affected by oxidation:
2005, January 15,

Titled, "Oxidation-induced ferritin turnover in microglial cells: role of proteasome." Dr. J. Mehlhase et. al., of the Neuroscience Research Center, Humboldt University, Berlin, Germany, reports that, "Highly oxidized protein aggregates accumulating in the brain during neurodegenerative diseases are often surrounded by microglia. Most of the microglial cells surrounding these plaques are activated and release a high amount of oxidizing species." *The team further relates that,* "In order to develop their toxic effects numerous oxidizing species need iron." *Reporting further the team relates that,* "Ferritin de novo synthesis was also severely affected by oxidation. This results in a decreased ferritin pool due to acute oxidative stress."

Stedman's Medical Dictionary describes ferritin as "**An iron-containing protein complex.**"

Thinking, about the above line, ferritin de novo [over again] synthesis was also severely affected by oxidation. <u>I have already shown in previous chapters that eugenol, methyl-eugenol and ethyl-vanillin are known oxidizers.</u>

Alzheimer's and, Iron induced oxidative stress:
2004. March

More evidence is presented titled, "Oxidative stress and redox-active iron in Alzheimer's disease." Dr. K. Honda and Associates, at the Institute of Pathology, Case Western University, Cleveland, Ohio, states that, "Many lines of evidence indicate that oxidative stress is one of the earliest events in the genesis of Alzheimer's disease [AD.] The team further states that, "Indeed both senile plaques and neurofibrillary tangles, the major pathological landmarks of AD, as well as neurons in the earliest stages of the disease show elevated iron deposition." In closing, Dr. Honda et al., reports that, "In this review, we consider the role of iron-induced oxidative stress as a key event in AD pathophysiology."

It is obvious to me, both from private research and testing on myself that iron needs to be replaced because the oxidizers eugenol, methyl-eugenol and ethyl-vanillin are oxidizing it out.

Remember in the manufactures [Rhodia] report that, "Vanillin is an interesting compound possessing both a phenolic and aldehydic group and is capable of undergoing a number of different types of chemical reactions." The key word here is phenolic or phenol. Keep phenol and vanillin in mind, I am working towards a point here.

Fenton's reagent:

From the Reference Library, "Peroxide Applications Industrial Wastewater" we find the chemical term, "Fenton's Reagent." It is stated in the introduction that, "Many metals have special oxygen transfer properties which improve the utility of hydrogen peroxide." It further states, "By far the most common of these is iron which, when used in the prescribed manner, results in the generation of highly reactive hydroxyl radicals [OH.] The reactivity of this system was first observed in 1894 by its inventor

H.J.H. Fenton." The report further states that, "Today Fenton's Reagent is used to treat a variety of industrial wastes containing a range of toxic organic compounds, Phenols, formaldehyde, BTEX, and complex wastes." On page three of the report, it is stated that, "In the absence of iron there is no evidence of hydroxyl radical formation when, for example, H_2O_2 is added to a phenolic wastewater [i.e., no reduction of phenol occurs] as the concentration of iron is increased, phenol removal accelerates."

Iron is needed to remove the phenol contained in the vanillin.

Webster's Dictionary defines Phenol as, "A corrosive poisonous crystalline acidic compound C6H5OH present in coal tar and wood tar that in dilute solution is used as a disinfectant." **Doesn't this partially describe ethyl-vanillin?**

Martin B. Hocking, of the University of Victoria, Department of Chemistry, Victoria, BC. relates in his paper, titled, "Journal of Chemical Education," that, "Vanillin production from the lignin-containing waste liquor obtained from acid sulfite pulping of wood began in North America in the mid 1930's. By 1981, one plant at Thorold, Ontario produced 60% of the contemporary world supply of vanillin." *Hocking goes on to say that,* "Today, however, whilst vanillin production from lignin is still practiced in Norway and a few other areas, all North American facilities using this process have closed, primarily for environmental reasons."

I want to make sure I have this right. The Government put a stop to extracting vanillin from the waste liquor obtained from acid sulfite pulping of wood because, these chemicals were polluting the environment?

It's ok to put ethyl-vanillin [an oxidizer] in our food, but not ok to pour these chemicals out onto the ground because, it's harmful to our environment?

Now, its ok to manufacture synthetic ethyl-vanillin at a chemical plant just be sure not to pour any of it on the ground.

Don't put it into metal containers either, because, the oxidation will eat holes in the metal.

Oh by the way, when you make ethyl-vanillin it will have two or three times the strength of just regular vanillin.

In my opinion, vanillin is not a memory problem for younger people who have a strong biochemical system. After all, ten and twenty year olds do not get Alzheimer's disease. Whether or not ethyl-vanillin can be a health problem in other areas, I have no way of knowing. I want to point out something here. Based on my findings, when the strength of vanillin is doubled or tripled its effects on my cognition are also doubled or tripled. When double emulsifiers were added, my memory was inhibited even further.

Zinc, copper and iron contribute to amyloid plaques, and Alzheimer's disease:

2004, *November, December*

Department of Neurology, National Creative Research Initiative Center for the Study of CNS Zinc, College of Medicine, University of Ulsan, Seoul 138-736 Korea D-Pharm Ltd., Kiryat Weizmann Science Park, Bldg. 7, P.O. Box 2313, Rehovot 76123, Israel reports in their work titled, "The lipophilic metal chelator DP-109 reduces amyloid pathology in brains of human beta-amyloid precursor protein transgenic mice." *In the report, first author, Dr. J.Y. Lee et al., states that,* "Metals such as zinc, copper and iron contribute to aggregation of amyloid-beta [abeta] protein and deposition of amyloid plaques in Alzheimer's disease [AD.]" *In summation, the team reports that,* "These results further support the hypothesis that endogenous metals are involved in the deposition of aggregated Abeta in brains of AD patients, and that metal chelators may be useful therapeutic agents in the treatment of AD."

See, metals are being oxidized!

Stedman's Medical Dictionary, describes Chelate as, "A chemical compound in the form of a heterocyclic ring, containing a metal ion attached by coordinate bonds to at least two non-metal ions."

Aren't these metals being oxidized by methyl-eugenol, ethyl-vanillin [artificial flavors] and then deposited in the beta amyloid plaque in the Alzheimer's brain?

There is no doubt in my mind, of how I came into possession of the *"six element"* replacement formula that reversed my Alzheimer's disease. I also know what I am supposed to do with this information. I have been studying practically day and night, seven days a week, for over 7 years now. I have been doing this to educate myself concerning the things involved in Alzheimer's dementia, so I can help end this disease.

"Faith can move mountains"

CHAPTER EIGHTEEN:
DREAMS

THE
"PROPHECY"
OF SIX NUMBERS

Understanding the odds

The odds are over 2.5 billion to 1 that this was just a random dream. Can you accept those kinds of odds that this dream of 6 numbers [6 elements] was a coincidence? I can't. Common sense alone dictates that 2.5 billion to 1 odds are just next to impossible.

To put that in perspective, would you bet on a horse which has odds of 100 to 1? How about a horse with odds of 2.5 billion to 1? These kinds of odds are just impossible to accept as a coincidence.

There are numerous events in the scriptures, where our Creator **caused a dream** to appear in order to help mankind.

One example is found in the book of Genesis in the Holy Bible.

Pharaoh, in a dream, received a vision, but no one could explain it. Joseph explained to Pharaoh, that God had given him a vision of a future event, to foretell a great tribulation. There would be seven years of plenty, followed by, seven years of famine. This allowed them to survive tremendous hardships, by storing up food.

Genesis 41:1-32.

Dreaming of Neurotransmitters:

Did God intervene here to help increase man's knowledge, **by causing a dream?**

The web site, http://faculty.washington.edu/chulder/chnt1.html

Relates information on the discovery of the Acetylcholine Neurotransmitter. The site says, "Back in 1920, an Austrian scientist named Otto Loewi, discovered the first neurotransmitter. In his experiment **[which came to him in a dream,]** he used two frog hearts. One heart [heart #1,] was still connected to the vagus nerve. Heart #1, was placed in a chamber that was filled with saline. This chamber was connected to a second chamber that contained heart #2." *The web site says,* "So fluid from chamber #1, was allowed to flow into chamber #2. Electrical stimulation of the vagus nerve [which was attached to heart #1] caused heart #1 to slow down. Loewi also observed that after a delay, heart *#2 also* slowed down." *The web site says,* "From this experiment Loewi hypothesized that electrical stimulation of the vagus nerve released a chemical into the fluid of chamber #1 that flowed into chamber #2. He called this chemical "Vagusstoff." We now know this chemical as the neurotransmitter called acetylcholine." The acetylcholine neurotransmitter is a major component of synaptic transmission. Choline needed for the acetylcholine neurotransmitter is in short supply in the Alzheimer's brain.

Was this another dream to help mankind?

Hindsight reveals that almost from the beginning, over twelve years ago, when I started to think about the cause and cure for the Alzheimer's disease, I had no idea of the amount of work that lay ahead of me. In what had started out as a way to help Mother with her Alzheimer's dementia became an obsession, of never ending day and night research of Alzheimer's.

The strange dream of *"six numbers and a large check"* was so real, I concluded the numbers would be the key and they might lead me to the check. I think the check was the motivator. It's all about stopping this horrible disease named Alzheimer's dementia and possibly finding answers for other neurodegenerative diseases.

The mysterious dream of
"Six Numbers."

This happened during 1993. If I had realized how important it was, I would have noted the hour and the day. I had probably been asleep an hour. This dream was very clear and very short. Unlike any dream I ever had before.

Six Numbers and a Check:

The man was dressed in a black business suit. His age appeared to be 45 years old to maybe mid 50's. He was five feet, seven inches, to maybe, five feet, ten inches tall. He handed me a very large check and said, "I'm giving you this check for these numbers." He then spoke these *"six numbers"* to me, *"3 - 7 - 9 - 11 - 14 - 26."* Immediately, I woke up and wrote them down. I thought, "Wow! What was this about?" Days later I thought, "Maybe I will win the lottery."

Reflecting back in time comes this scenario. Mother told me that when I was eight or nine months old, she and dad were trying to get me to start walking. Nothing seemed to work. Then Dad got an idea. He reached in his pocket and pulled out a silver dollar [not an uncommon coin in 1935.] Mom said, that when he held it up, I stood up and walked over and got it.

Thinking about the check in the dream, motivation comes to mind. Something else here comes to mind, why did I wake up with the numbers riveted in my thoughts even more so than the numbers on the check? Was this so I would not forget them?

As time went by, something else was happening, I was becoming able to smell certain chemicals in my food. I have thought many times about this. When I eat food or drink liquids that have the chemical additives of artificial flavors combined with emulsifiers in them, and, I am at risk for Alzheimer's, which means, I am not protecting myself by replacing the *"six elements,"* I can smell these chemicals on my skin. I can spend 30 minutes in a room, leave and come back in an hour or so and I can smell this strange odor in the room from when I was there before.

The first time I smelled it was about one year before Mom died, and about one year before I realized this disease was now coming after me. When I entered the care facility that morning, I smelled it in the air and near my mother. I now, had the ability to smell a strange foreign odor that the body emits when the body can no longer process these combined chemical food and drink additives. The process of an elimination diet helped, but, it was the fact that I was able to smell the strange foreign odor that enabled me to figure out that it was methyl-eugenol, ethyl-vanillin [artificial flavors] combined with propylene-glycol [emulsifier] that I ingested from foods and drinks which were causing my memory problems.

I believe in Creation and I try to remember to be respectful of all the world religions. There are so many different ones. Each and everyone will swear they are correct in their beliefs. It is for this reason that I try to keep an open mind concerning my faith.

I believe when we were created he gave us free will to reason and make our own decisions. I believe we are tested daily. How strong is your faith? Do you believe God knows how to cure the Alzheimer's disease? In a way, this book is a test. If you need a little help to believe, just consider the odds [over two billion to one] of having a dream representing *"six very important elements"* that are definitely involved in the Alzheimer's disease.

God truly does work miracles!

After the strange dream, I had started to play the lottery using the *"six numbers"* that were in the dream. I continued to play the numbers in the lottery for about 6 years.

Motivation is a very strong incentive. Although the dream happened over 12 years ago, it provided enough motivation that I am still pursuing this to its completion.

If you want to see an extreme example of motivation, read Chapter 9 in *"The book of Acts"* from the *"The Holy Bible."*

Six years of searching:

Over the next six years, I spent an enormous amount of time trying to use these numbers to identify their purpose. This search lead me through lottery numbers, trying to identify the unabomber, even to try and locate the missing millions in two armored car robberies for the rewards by using the numbers as phone numbers and addresses. The numbers even form a social security number.

As a former Commercial Pilot, I even explored geographical latitude and longitude locations using the *"six numbers"* to try and track the culprits in the two armored car robberies.

I discovered there were four locations on the planet these numbers could identify. I thought possibly, one of these fellows had gone to Brazil and the other to the Azores. I will not go into detail why I thought that. I ordered aviation charts from Jeppeson and spent weeks working on them.

I even had to work my way through "Fiber Optics research" to try and define the purpose of the *"six numbers."* Have you ever heard of the lithium ion generator? [Think number 3, lithium.] Silicon is also involved in fiber optics. [Silicon is number 14.] This probably took me a month or two to realize the answers I was looking for did not lie in fiber optics.

Looking back, I can see where the road block was in my search for answers and my thoughts drift back to that December day in 1950. It was Christmas vacation, and my family was moving from Everglades City on Florida's West coast, to Miami on Florida's East coast. I was 15 years old and in the 10th grade of high school. As Mom and I drove east towards Miami on highway 41, the old Tamiami Trail that connected the East and West coast of Florida, I remember saying, "Mom, I think I want to quit school, I'm bored." She asked, "Are you sure?" I replied, "Yes," and that was that. I joined the labor force and became a third generation craftsman.

There was absolutely nothing in my 49 year work history that would give me a clue for defining these *"six numbers."*

I was employed for awhile as an international corporate pilot, flying heavy 4 engine aircraft. I would call this professional employment. However, even this did not bring me into contact with the one thing that would help me solve this mystery.

At the time of the dream, what I did not understand was the significance of the numbers. By now, Mother had started to develop advanced Alzheimer's symptoms. At that time, I was not smart enough, to know what the numbers were really for yet. Six years had now gone by and I was not one step closer to solving this mysterious dream.

Then one day, while driving down the street and thinking about the *"six numbers"* in the dream, I thought maybe I need to look elsewhere. After all, I had used these numbers for six years playing lotteries and searching through other things with no success. Then I started to think about gold. For over twenty years markets and commodities were something I had studied as a hobby. Let me see, gold has a symbol of Au. Somewhere, I had heard everything had an atomic number, so off to the used bookstore I went.

"Say, do you have any information on Atomic numbers?" I asked. "You mean, the Periodic Table of Elements" the book store manager said.

"Bingo."

I bought a complete set of McGraw-Hill Encyclopedias of Science and Technology along with other Medical books. Like the Funk and Wagnall's-Atlas of the Body, the Vitamin Book-Bantam Books. The Mosby Medical Encyclopedia, Dr. Wright's book of Nutritional Therapy, Biology-Cliffs quick review and Chemistry-Cliffs quick review to use for research.

Over the next five years, many more books would be purchased in this quest for knowledge and to research with. I would spend many long nights reading and looking up definitions of medical terms published in neuroscientist's research papers. In order to understand this disease, I needed more knowledge, I needed more education, and I needed more books.

One thing is paramount here:

If I would have stayed in school, I would have been exposed to the *"Periodic Table of Elements"* in chemistry, and had the answer sooner and Mom might still be alive. There was nothing wrong with Mother's physical health. Alzheimer's took her life and took her away from her family and friends.

This discovery of what the numbers might mean appeared when I was about one year into my process of elimination diet to try and discover what was causing this cognitive impairment in me. I was developing the same memory problems that caused Mothers death, Alzheimer's disease.

I would spend day and night for the next twelve months researching these elements and how the body used them, to see if these *"six elements"* did indeed work to stop this mental impairment that had started on me, just like it did on Mother.

When I first started to convert the *"six numbers"* from the dream into *"six elements"* from the Periodic Table, the only atomic element I recognized was iron [Fe] number 26. After many more months of continual research, I began to understand how important the other *"five numbers"* [elements] are to our mental health and memory. I remember when I became aware that I had finally solved the meaning of these *"six numbers,"* I felt so blessed. Now maybe I would not have to die with Alzheimer's disease like Mother did.

Mother had described these very same symptoms to me. The same problems, confusion, short term memory loss, disorientation and at times not being able to think progressively. Problems with numbers. This Alzheimer's disease had set its sights on me.

These *"six numbers,"* when converted to the *"Periodic Table of Atomic Elements,"* provide the compound to keep my brain cells free of plaque, but, there is much more involved here than just amyloid plaque.

After several more months of testing on myself, I was able to completely reverse the cognitive impairment and dementia that had affected my memory by replacing the "six elements" *on a regular basis.*

In Chapter 17, it is plain to see that the 6 elements [6 numbers] are directly involved in Alzheimer's dementia.

<u>Following this Chapter, dated March 28, 1998, is a copy of one of the last lottery tickets I bought using the</u> "six numbers." **I finally realized the purpose for the numbers. It had nothing to do with the lottery, and I haven't played those lottery numbers since.**

<u>Also included at the end of this Chapter is a display of the</u> "Periodic Table of Elements."

Regarding the "Periodic Table of Elements," *P.W. Atkins says, in his book titled, Periodic Kingdom,* "Welcome to the periodic kingdom. This is a land of the imagination, but it is closer to reality than it appears to be. This is the kingdom of the chemical elements, the substances from which everything is made." *Atkins further relates that,* "These elements are the basis of the air, the oceans, and the earth itself. We stand on the elements, we eat the elements, we are the elements. Because our brains are made up of elements, even our opinions are, in a sense, properties of the elements and hence inhabitants of the kingdom."

In the early 1800's, atomic elements were still being discovered but were not organized into a table, as we know them today. Chemists were trying to find a way to accomplish this organization. The man who figured this out was a chemist named Dmitri Ivanovitch Mendeleev.

Another Dream to help mankind?

P. W. Atkins, relates in his book that, "Mendeleev looked a little like the mad monk of Rasputin and had a reputation to match." *Atkins further relates that,* "It is said that during a brief nap in the course of writing a textbook of chemistry, for which he was struggling with the problem of the order in which to introduce the elements, **he had a dream.** When he awoke, he set out his chart, in virtually its final form."

"Periodic Kingdom" by P. W. Atkins, Is an excellent book!

Today, scientists know that matter is represented in the *"Periodic Table of Elements."* The Periodic Table is constructed of elements which are made up of atoms. Atoms contain a nucleus in the center, made up of neutrons and protons. The exception is hydrogen, having a nucleus of only one proton. The protons carry a positive electrical charge. The neutrons carry no electrical charge.

The protons and neutrons are held together in the center of the nucleus by a means scientists refer to as the strong force. A cloud of electrons surrounds the nucleus. These electrons carry a negative electrical charge. A particular element in the Periodic Table assumes its place by the number of protons in its nucleus.

The element hydrogen has one proton in its nucleus and it is represented as number one in the Periodic Table. It has one electron in the outer shell that is negatively charged. This equals the one proton that carries a positive charge. Since the negative and positive charges are equal, this is called an electrically neutral atom.

When an atom gains or loses electrons it is referred to as an "ion," and becomes electrically charged.

When an atom loses electrons, then it has a positive charge. Positive charged atoms are referred to as "Cations."

When an atom gains electrons, it has a negative charge. Negatively charged atoms are called Anions.

Yes, there is indeed a definite mathematical arrangement of the atomic elements in the Periodic Table.

Considering that all existence is constructed in such a marvelous order and pondering the wonderful manner in which our bodies are constructed and function, it is hard to imagine there are those who choose not to believe in a Supreme Creator.

Father, we thank you for
All you have given us.
Amen.

My Alzheimer's symptoms are gone.
The same kind of symptoms that
eventually caused my mothers death.

The element replacement along
with a restricted diet, restored
my memory and normal cognition.

After years of Alzheimer's research and
self testing, here is my question,
isn't this disease caused by a
deficiency of vitamins and 6 atomic elements?

A three year process of elimination
diet allowed me to discover how
this disease manifests itself.

I urge you to read this book
and then, discuss it with your doctor.

www.zapalzheimers.com

The Periodic Table of the Elements

LITHIUM SODIUM NITROGEN SILICON FLUORINE IRON

1	2	3	4	5	6	7	8	9	10	11	12	13	14	15	16	17	18
1 H																	2 He
3 Li	4 Be											5 B	6 C	7 N	8 O	9 F	10 Ne
11 Na	12 Mg											13 Al	14 Si	15 P	16 S	17 Cl	18 Ar
19 K	20 Ca	21 Sc	22 Ti	23 V	24 Cr	25 Mn	26 Fe	27 Co	28 Ni	29 Cu	30 Zn	31 Ga	32 Ge	33 As	34 Se	35 Br	36 Kr
37 Rb	38 Sr	39 Y	40 Zr	41 Nb	42 Mo	43 Tc	44 Ru	45 Rh	46 Pd	47 Ag	48 Cd	49 In	50 Sn	51 Sb	52 Te	53 I	54 Xe
55 Cs	56 Ba	57 La [1]	72 Hf	73 Ta	74 W	75 Re	76 Os	77 Ir	78 Pt	79 Au	80 Hg	81 Tl	82 Pb	83 Bi	84 Po	85 At	86 Rn
87 Fr	88 Ra	89 Ac [2]	104 Rf	105 Db	106 Sg	107 Bh	108 Hs	109 Mt	110 Uun	111 Uuu	112 Uub		114 Uuq		116 Uuh		118 Uuo

[1]	58 Ce	59 Pr	60 Nd	61 Pm	62 Sm	63 Eu	64 Gd	65 Tb	66 Dy	67 Ho	68 Er	69 Tm	70 Yb	71 Lu
[2]	90 Th	91 Pa	92 U	93 Np	94 Pu	95 Am	96 Cm	97 Bk	98 Cf	99 Es	100 Fm	101 Md	102 No	103 Lr

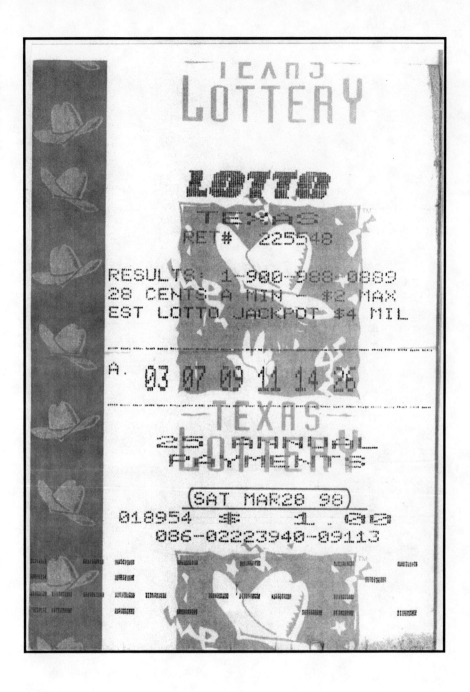

TEXAS
LOTTERY

LOTTO
TEXAS
RET# 225548

RESULTS: 1-900-988-0889
28 CENTS A MIN — $2 MAX
EST LOTTO JACKPOT $4 MIL

A. 03 07 09 11 14 26

TEXAS
25 ANNUAL
PAYMENTS

SAT MAR28 98
018954 $ 1.00
086-02223940-09113

BIBLIOGRAPHY

Neuroresearchers:

Alvarez, Dr. G. and Associates, *Re: Accumulation of the beta-amyloid characterizes Alzheimer's: 2002, June, www.pubmed.gov 12180271.*

Aquilano, Dr. K. and Associates, *Re: Cross talk between copper, zinc and the SOD mutant: 2003, June, www.pubmed.gov 12753090.*

Arlt, Dr. S. et al., *Re: Oxidation and Aging: December 2001, www.pubmed.gov 11828885.*

Behl, Dr. C. and Dr. B. Moosmann, *Re: disease involves neuronal cell dysfunction: 2002, March-April, www.pubmed.gov 12033440.*

Belles, Dr. M. et al., *Re: Silicon reduces gastrointestinal aluminum absorption: 1998, www.pubmed.gov 9651136.*

Blass, Dr. J. P., *Re: Reactive nitrogen species: 2001, December, www.pubmed.gov 11746411.*

Boje, Dr. K. M., *Re: Reactive nitrogen oxide species. Neuroprotection or neurotoxicity: 2004, January, www.pubmed.gov 14766406.*

Calabrese, Dr. V. and Associates, *Re: Reactive nitrogen species involved in neurodegeneration:*
2004, May-June, *www.pubmed.gov 15341181.*

Chobpattana, Dr. W. et al., *R.: "Kinetics of interaction of **vanillin** with amino acids and peptides in model systems. The reaction rate of vanillin-amino acids/peptides were accelerated as temperature increased." www.pubmed.gov 10995286*

Dravid, S.M. Dr: et al., *Re: voltage-gated sodium channels: 2004, May, www. pubmed.gov 15086530.*

Edwardson, Dr. J. A. and Associates, *Re: High concentrations of aluminum found in plaques: 1986, www.pubmed.gov 3743229.*

Elyaman, Dr. W. and Associates, *Re: Lithium inhibits increase in tau phosphorylation: 2002, May, www.pubmed.gov 12065646.*

Emerit, Dr. J. et al., *Re: Reactive nitrogen species, oxidative stress and protein misfolding: 2004, January, www.pubmed.gov 14739060.*

Espey, Dr. M. G. and Associates, *Re: Reactive nitrogen oxide species: 2002, May, www.pubmed.gov 12076975.*

Fletcher, Dr. Robert and Dr. Kathleen Fairfield,
Re: "Low levels of folic acid and vitamins B-6 and B-12, are a risk factor for heart disease." www.pubmed.gov 12069675.

Granados-Perez, Dr. and Associates, *Re: Ultra trace elements are currently being studied: 2002, www.pubmed.gov 12166372.*

Green, Dr. Robert C. et al., *Re: Statin Drugs May Lower Risk of Alzheimer's, www.pubmed.gov 12454325.*

Grimes, Dr. C.A. and Dr. R.S. Jope, *Re: Lithium, a selective inhibitor of GSK-3 beta 2001, November, www.pubmed.gov 11527574.*

Grundman, Dr. M. et al., *Re: Oxidative damage in the Alzheimer's brain: 2002, May, www.pubmed.gov 12133201.*

Haynes, Dr. C. M. et al., *Re: Misfolded proteins lead to cellular damage and death: 2004, September 10, www. pubmed.gov 15350220.*

Honda, Dr. K. and Associates, *Re: Alzheimer's and Iron induced oxidative stress, 2004, March, www.pubmed.gov 15105265.*

Ischiropoulos, Dr. H., *Re: Reactive nitrogen species inhibits fibril formation: 2003, June, www.pubmed.gov 12846977.*

Kontush, Dr. A. et al., *Re: Oxidation, Lipids and Lipoproteins: 2001, August, www.pubmed.gov 11461772.*

Kutscher, Dr. C., *"Notes on Chapter 4, Carlson Psychopharmacology,"* C. Kutscher, Spring 2001, *http://psychweb.syr.edu/psy323/notes/NotesCh4323.htm*

Lee, Dr. J.Y. et al., *Re: Zinc, copper and iron contribute to amyloid plaques and Alzheimer's disease: 2004, November- December, www. pubmed.gov 15465629.*

Mehlhase, Dr. J. et al., *Re: Ferritin synthesis severely affected by oxidation: 2005, January 15, www.pubmed.gov 15607911.*

Moreno-Sanchez, Dr. C. et al., *Re: Oxidative Stress: 2004, March,* *www.pubmed.gov* *14988463.*

Paris, Dr. Daniel et al., *Re: Statins block the* *vasoconstrictive effect of the A-beta protein.* *www.pubmed.gov* *11888511.*

Phiel, Dr. C.J. and Associates, *Re: Lithium blocks accumulation of* *abeta peptides: 2003, May,* *www.pubmed.gov* *12761548.*

Rivera, Dr. Victor, *Re: elevated temperature,* *slows down the conduction of the nerve impulses.*

Ryder, Dr. J. and Associates, *Re: Lithium reduces abeta production:* *2003, December,* *www.pubmed.gov* *14651959.*

Senatorov, Dr. V. V. et al., *Re: Lithium reduces neuron damage: 2004,* *April,* *www.pubmed.gov* *14702090.*

Tappel, Dr. A., *Re: Free radical lipid peroxidation,* 2004, *www.* *pubmed.gov* *15193357.*

Vieira, Dr. E. P., Dr. H. Hermel and Dr. H.

Mohwald, *Re: Fluorinated alcohols can refold the beta-conformation:* *2003, January,* *www.pubmed.gov* *12535605.*

Wrona, Dr. M.Z. et al., *Re: Oxidation by reactive nitrogen species:* *2003, April,* *www.pubmed.gov* *12703966.*

Recommended Reference Books:

Alcamo, Edward I. Ph.D. *Biology,* *[Cliff Notes Inc. 1993.]*

American Heritage, *Stedman's* Medical Dictionary, *[Marion* *Severynse, editor, Houghton Mifflin, Co. 2002.]*

Atkins, P.W., *Periodic Kingdom,* *[Basic Books, 1995.]*

Cranton, Elmer M. M.D., *Bypassing Bypass* *Surgery,* *[Hampton Roads 2001.]*

Dennerll, Jean Tannis BS, CMA., *Medical Terminology Made* *Easy,* *[Thomson Delmar Learing, 2003.]*

Dox, Ida G. PH.D., B. John Melloni PH.D., Gilbert M. Eisner M.D., June L. Melloni PH.D.

The Harper Collins Illustrated Medical Dictionary, *[Harper Collins* *2001.]*

Eby, Denise and Robert B. Horton, *Physical Science,* *[Macmillan* *Publishing Co. 1988.]*

Fox, Barry Ph.D., *Foods to Heal By,* *[Lynn Sonberg Book Associates,* *1996.]*

Funk & Wagnalls Atlas of the Body, *[Rand McNally and Co. 1992.]*

Goldberg, Dr. Burton, *Studies in Alternative Medicine, [Future Medicine Publishing Company, 1993.]*

Herbert, Victor M.D. and Genell J. Subak-Sharpe, *Total Nutrition, [St. Martin's Press 1994.]*

Jablonski, Dr. Stanley, *Dictionary of Medical Acronyms and Abbreviations, [Hanley and Belfus 2001.]*

Kapit, Wynn, Robert I. Macey and Esmail Meisami, *Physiology Coloring Book, [Addison Wesley Longman, 2000.]*

Lieberman, Dr. Shari and Nancy Bruning, *Real Vitamin and Mineral Book, [Avery, 1997.]*

McGraw-Hill Encyclopedias of Science and Technology, *defines clove, 7th Edition, page 39, [McGraw-Hill, 1992.]*

Medina, John Ph.D., *What you need to know about Alzheimer's, [New Harbinger Publications, 1999.]*

Merck Manual of Medical Information, Home Edition 1997, *[Robert Berkow, M.D., editor in chief, Merck Research Labotatories, 1997.]*

Merriam-Webster's Collegiate Dictionary, Tenth Edition, *[Merriam-Webster Inc. 2001.]*

Mosby Medical Encyclopedia, Revised Edition, *[Walter D. Glanze, managing editor, 1992]*

Murray, Michael T. N. D., *Encyclopedia of Nutritional Supplements [Prima Publishing. 1997.]*

Nathan, Harold D. Ph.D., *Chemistry, [Cliff Notes Inc., 1993.]*

O'Conner, Rod, *[Fundamentals of Chemistry, 1977.]*

Pressman, Alan H. D.C., Ph.D., C.C.N., *Vitamins and Minerals, [Macmilln Inc., 1997.]*

Siegfried, Dr. Donna Rae, *Anatomy & Physiology for Dummies, [Wiley Publishing Inc., 2002.]*

Smith, Patricia B., Mary Mitchell Kenan PsyD, and Mark Edwin Kunik M.D. MPH., *Alzheimer's for Dummies, [Wiley Publishing Co., 2004.]*

Stansfield, William D., Jaime S. Colome, and Raul J. Cano, *Molecular and Cell Biology, [McGraw-Hill, 1996.]*

Stryer, Dr. Lubert, *Biochemistry,* *[W. H. Freeman and Company,1981.]*

Taylor, Dr. Richard, *Alzheimer's, from the Inside Out,* [Health Professionals Press, 2007.]

Waller, Robert R. M.D. *Mayo Clinic Family Health Boo , [William Morrow and Co. 1996.]*

Web Sites:

"Melatonin may be the most important anti-oxidant supplement you can take."

http://www.lef.org/prod_desc/mela01.htm

"**Ethyl vanillin** is soluble in alcohol," Rhodia,

http://www.food.us.rhodia.com/brochures/romexpvn/page4.asp

"Kinetics of interaction of **vanillin** with amino acids and peptides in model systems."

http://www.confex.com/ift/99annual/abstracts/3603.htm

"The number of people with dementia is rising quickly."

http://www.Alz.co.uk/alzwp.htm

"Seven ways to open the Blood brain barrier."

http://faculty.washington.edu/chudler/bbb.html

"**Eugenol** known by the Iupac [International Union of Pure and Applied Chemistry] name."

http://www.scorecard.org/chemical-.../consumer-products.tcl? edf_substance_id=97%2d53%2d

"Eugenol oil overdoses; poisonous ingredient actions." *http://Webmd/Lycos-article-eugenol oil overdose*

"Eugenol, Statement of Hazards. Caution! Skin and eye irritation. Liver damage." *www.ehs.cornell.edu/lrs/labels/Eugenol.html,*

"**Eugenol;** 5.3 human data.

No case report or epidemiological study of the carcinogenicity of eugenol to humans was available." *http://193.51164.11/htdocs/monographs/vol36/eugenol.html*

"The destructive effects of **propylene glycol- ethyl vanillin** on metals." *Oxidation photograph, www.zapalzheimers.com*

165

"**Eugenol**, occurs widely as a component of essential oils."
http://193.51.164.11/htdocs/monographs/vol36/eugenol.html

"**Vanillin** is an interesting compound, possessing both a phenolic and aldehydic group."

http://www.food.us.rhodia.com/brochures/epv/page17.asp

"Alzheimer's disease ranks fourth in the cause of deaths among adults." *http://www.downtownagusta.com/alzheimersstatistics.htm*

"There is no generally accepted source for an authoritative list of chemicals that are recognized to cause neurotoxicity."

http://www.scorecard.org/health-effects/references.tcl? Short hazard name=neuro 10/21/01.

"We are a manufacture from China. We produce and export food additive vanillin, other **vanillin**, **ethyl vanillin,** etc."

www.tradezone.com/tradesites/girasole.html

"**Eugenol**; chemical health hazard. Suspected gastrointestinal or liver toxicant, neurotoxicant."

http://www.scorecard.org/chemicalprofiles/summary.tcl?edf_substance_id=97-53-0

"**Eugenol**; is used in the production of iso-eugenol for the manufacture of vanillin."

http://ntpdb.niehs.nih.gov/ntp_reports/ntp_chem_h&s/ntp_chem9/radian97-53-0.tx

"**Vanillin** synonyms."

http://chemcourses.ucsd.edu/coursepages/uglabs/msds/vanillin-info.html

"**Vanillic acid;** Material Safety Data Sheet, Handling and storage of vanillic acid."

http://www.alfa.com/cgibin/odc_webcat/jump.cgi?File=msds/a12074.html

"**Vanillin.**

Containers should be closed and kept away from light, heat and moisture. It is recommended to avoid using iron or steel containers."

http://www.food.us.rhodia.com/datasheets/template1.asp? PID=222

"**Vanillin** can react with iron to form a pinkish-colored compound."

http://www.foodproductdesign.com/archive/1998/0898cs.html

"**Extra pure ethyl vanillin** is 2.6 times stronger in flavor than vanillin."

http://www.food.us.rhodia.com/brochures/romexpvn/page2.asp

"**Eugenol** is highly toxic in concentrated form."

http://darkwing.uoregon.edu/~sshapiro/pemphigus/phenolics.html

"The National Institute of Standards and Technology, [NIST]**O-vanillin,** This chemical is incompatible with iron, zinc, ferric chloride, and potassium permanganate. Located on page 2 dated, November 22, 2000." *http://webbook.nist.gov/cgi/cbook.cgi? Id=c148538&units=si [2-hydroxy-3-methoxybenzaldehyde.]*

"**Ethyl vanillic acid** has been identified in the urine of humans known to have ingested vanilla-flavored foodstuffs."

http://www.inchem.org/documents/jecfa/jecmono/v35j07.htm

"**Vanillin,** harmful if swallowed. University of California, S. D. Chemistry & Biochemistry," *http://chemcourses.ucsd.edu/coursepages/ uglabs/msds/vanillin. -Info.htm, page 2 and 3, November 13, 2000.*

"**Eugenol,** an experimental carcinogen and tumorigen. Human mutagenic data. A human skin irritant."

http://ntpdb.niehs.nih.gov/ntp reports/ntp chem h&s/ntp chem9radian 97-53-0.txt May 23, 2000

"Toxicity of **vanillin** to lettuce using water with 650 plus **or** minus 30 mg/1 produced a 50% reduction in germination." *http://www. inchem.org/documents/sids/sids/sids5b06.html*

"Few metabolism studies had been carried out on **ethyl vanillin**."

http://www.inchem.org/documents/jecfa/jecmono/v35je07.htm

"**Emulsifiers,** Small quantities, large effect."

http://www.lci-koeln.de/498engl.html, February 16, 2001.

Lists Stabilizers.

http://www.pacifichealth.com/gras list.htm.

Lists emulsifying agents.

http://www.pacifichealth.com/gras list.htm.

"**Eugenol** was reported to inhibit respiration in vitro in mitochondria."

http://www.inchem.org/documents/jecfa/jecmono/v17je10htm

"Clove oil, like all spice is 60-90 percent **eugenol.**"

http://vitawise.com/clove.htm

"Numerous synthetic and natural compounds mutate cellular DNA, and cause cancer cells to form."

http://www.lef.org/prod_desc/mela01.htm

Describes Aluminum.

http:// www.merriam-webster.com

"Aluminum is known to be a significant cross-linking agent that acts to immobilize reactive molecules."

http://www.connectcorp.net/~trufax/mercury/alum.html

"Trace elements are also known as micronutrients."

http://www.anyvitamins.com/trace-elements-info.htm

"The total trace elements in our bodies would barley fill a thimble, but that thimble full is needed to sustain life."

http://www.traceminerals.com/about.html

"Like your body, it only lights up with ionic trace minerals."

http://www.traceminerals.com/ions.html

"The nitrogen cycle is one of the most important processes in nature for living organisms."

http://pearl1.lanl.gov/periodic/elements/7.html

"Discovery of the Acetylcholine Neurotransmitter." Dr. Otto Loewi, Austrian scientist.

www./faculty.washington.edu/chulder/chnt1.html

"Life is essentially nothing more than a variety of biochemical reactions." Degussa Health and Nutrition Facts.

http://www.degussa-health-nutrition.com/ degussa/html/e/health/eng/kh/i4.htm

Health and Nutrition:

"High-calorie diets loaded with fats may spell trouble for people with a genetic predisposition for the memory-robbing Alzheimer's disease. "

Reuters-Health, Wednesday, August 14, 2002.

"Motion to list **methyl-eugenol** as reasonably anticipated to be a human carcinogen passed by a vote of 9 yes to 1 no. The National Toxicology Program [NTP.]" *Public Health Service Department of*

Health and Human Services. *Federal Register: volume. 66 no. 43. Notices. Pages 13334 - 13338, March 5, 2001.*

"Focus: Multiple Sclerosis, [MS] cool fashion."

Deborah Mann Lake, Houston Chronicle, page 20a, titled, Tuesday, October 2, 2001.

"**Vanillin:** Synthetic flavoring from spent sulfite liquor." *Dr. Martin B. Hocking J. Chem. Educ. 1997 74 1055.*

"One neurologist stated that 95% of the people he diagnoses with Alzheimer's are not even tested." *Dr. Richard Taylor, Houston and Southwest Texas Chapter of the Alzheimer's Association.*

"Suffered with Alzheimer's, became lucid."

Dr. Joe Graedon and Dr. Teresa Graedon, Houston Chronicle, Friday, Nov. 2, 2001.

"The first actual description of ethyl-vanillin occurs in a German patent, registered by Schering in 1894." *Rhodia, "**Extra Pure Ethyl Vanillin**," April 2, 2002.*

"The Aztecs used **vanillin** as a flavoring and it was brought to Europe by Cortez in about 1520."

The University of New South Whales, Sidney, Australia, School of Chemistry.

"Iron Deficiency May Contribute To Alzheimer Damage." *Merritt McKinney, New York Reuters Health.*

"Fenton's Reagent, Re: "Iron- catalyzed Hydrogen Peroxide." page three, Peroxide Applications Industrial Wastewater.*

Index

A

abeta production 133, 163
acetylcholine neurotransmitter xx, 3,
    10, 34, 114, 120, 130, 139, 150
Advil 7
age-weakened 11, 15, 17, 59, 73, 75,
    76, 79, 88, 121, 129
alcohol xx, 20, 21, 45, 49, 52, 53, 56,
    57, 61, 69, 74, 77, 79, 89, 95,
    101, 102, 104, 120, 124, 165
aldehyde 46, 64, 68
aldehydic 55, 56, 146, 166
Aleve 7, 141
Alois Alzheimer 9, 12, 13
Aluminum 17, 93, 94, 115, 120, 142,
    143, 144, 168
Alzheimer's 103
Alzheimer genes 79
amino acid xx, 35, 36, 37, 44, 45, 51,
    85, 130, 134, 136, 141
Amyloidosis 57
amyloid beta 40 53
amyloid beta 42 53
amyloid precursor protein 53, 78,
    133, 148
anti-freeze 73, 83
antioxidant 19, 33, 86, 130
apoe4 90
argon 56
aspartame 47, 94
Astrodome 23
atherosclerosis 19
Atomic numbers 154
autopsies 94
axon 34, 43
a miracle 31

B

bakery products 68, 74, 83, 88, 122,
    130
baking products 81
beta amyloid plaque 10, 21, 34, 57,
    76, 119, 143, 148
biochemical xv, 1, 2, 10, 11, 13, 15,
    17, 21, 32, 33, 39, 41, 42, 47,
    51, 57, 58, 59, 60, 66, 67, 68,
    69, 70, 72, 73, 74, 76, 80, 81,
    88, 100, 101, 110, 111, 113,
    114, 121, 122, 125, 126, 129,
    130, 141, 144, 147, 168
biochemical defense system 10, 32,
    33, 57, 59, 60, 68, 73, 74, 76,
    101, 111
biochemical reactions xv, 2, 11, 15,
    39, 42, 51, 76, 125, 126, 130,
    141, 168
biochemical synthesis 141
Biotin 50
blocked arteries 20, 135
Blood Brain Barrier 25, 26
book of Genesis 149
brain fibers 10, 11, 34
brake fluids 17, 73, 83

C

calcium 111, 135, 138
California 6, 77, 116, 117, 131, 167
calories 66, 67, 73, 87, 88, 97, 100,
    102, 103, 122, 124
Calorie Restriction 88
cancer 20, 40, 87, 90, 168
Cancer cells 91
candy lover 103
canonical 45

oxidation xv, 16, 17, 40, 47, 49, 63, 67, 93, 117, 123, 125, 126, 130, 131, 134, 135, 136, 145, 147, 162

oxidative stress 67, 111, 123, 125, 130, 136, 138, 145, 146, 162

oxidized nitrogen 136, 138, 139

oxidizer 13, 17, 47, 60, 83, 112, 121, 122, 123, 130, 144, 147

oxidizing metals 125

P

pain relievers 26

Pantothenic acid 50, 124

Parkinsons disease 137

pathogenesis xix, 16, 126, 131, 136, 143

Pennsylvania 7, 133, 137

pentalysine 47

Periodic Kingdom 155, 156, 163

Periodic Table of Elements 17, 18, 28, 74, 109, 112, 123, 129, 132, 135, 141, 144, 154, 155, 156

pharmaceuticals 65, 81

Phenol 55, 62, 147

phenyl 20

phenylalanine 47

photochemistry 16

photoemission 16

photolysis 16

Photo Dynamics 16

pineal gland 57, 58, 85, 86, 89

Plaques 34

polarized 2, 27

potassium 27, 35, 75, 76, 110, 111, 114, 115, 142, 167

pray ix, 70, 124

Presenilin 12

prion-based disease 140

prion protein 78

PROPHECY 149

propylene 15, 16, 17, 19, 33, 53, 66, 67, 73, 74, 83, 97, 114, 123, 124, 130, 141, 144, 152, 165

propylene-glycol 16, 17, 19, 33, 67, 73, 74, 83, 114, 123, 124, 141, 144, 152

Prozac 141

Pyridoxine 50, 124

R

radiation 11, 16, 57, 58, 77, 144

radioactive elements 99

reactive nitrogen species 136, 137, 138, 163

red blood cells 50

Red Cross toothache medicine 82, 121

research xiii, xvii, 1, 4, 5, 6, 11, 13, 15, 25, 30, 46, 49, 50, 52, 57, 58, 69, 71, 77, 80, 87, 90, 97, 98, 101, 107, 108, 111, 116, 117, 126, 129, 130, 131, 139, 140, 143, 145, 146, 150, 153, 154, 155, 157

retina 57, 89

rheumatoid arthritis 57

Rhodia 13, 53, 56, 66, 67, 68, 146, 165, 169

Riboflavin 49, 124

ribonucleic acid 45, 79

S

Schizophrenia 37

science 5, 10, 16, 21, 129

Scientific research 58, 69

scientists 25, 55, 88, 97, 156

senile plaques 34, 146

senility 21, 90

serotonin xx, 35, 36, 45, 51, 85, 130, 136, 141

silica and silicates 142

silicon 17, 99, 106, 108, 115, 120, 122, 123, 130, 143, 144, 145

Silicon reduces aluminum 143

six elements 21, 32, 33, 44, 69, 70, 74, 91, 98, 105, 106, 109, 113, 114, 123, 139, 151, 155

Printed in the United States
110540LV00004B/121/P

9 781434 318237